VICTORY Over Sickness and Pain

New insights and experiences to get and stay free

Chuck Schiappacasse

 Author may be reached at (847) 635-7636
ISBN 0-9635913-3-9
Cover design by Steve Vanides
Printed in the United States of America

The following standard abbreviations are indicated when other versions are quoted: KJV for the King James Version and NIV for the New International Version.

Also by Chuck Schiappacasse:

"God Heals Today", 1993, Second Printing, 1995
"God's Health Care Plan", 1995

CONTENTS

About the Author

Chuck Schiappacasse is a free-lance writer. Along with his wife, Faye, he's on the volunteer staff of Good News Church in Des Plaines, Illinois. Chuck and Faye head nursing home and door-to-door outreach ministries of the church. They are also active in prison ministry and host a home bible fellowship for the church.

In their more than fourteen years of ministry, the Schiappacasses have been involved in a growing number of healings and deliverances. A large percentage of the cases noted in this book are taken from their experiences.

Chuck's first book,"God Heals Today", features over 70 medically-confirmed cases of divine healing. His following book, "God's Health Care Plan, " includes both physical and emotional healings. These books are available in or through bookstores internationally. They can also be ordered by calling 1-800-760-BOOK.

FOREWORD

It was the weekend before the 1996 New Hampshire Primary. The New England city was bustling with activity. President Clinton would speak that afternoon. During the morning , a particular local radio station was preparing to broacast the speech live.

That same morning, I was scheduled to interview by phone on that station about my book, "God Heals Today". The host was uptight. During a commercial break, he agreed to prayer. I commanded spirits of stress and tension to leave him in the name of Jesus Christ. He noticed a difference. He said he felt like sitting down. Back on the air, he told the audience a little of what had happened.

At a home bible study, a mother and young-adult son complained of inordinate perspiring. This problem had been recurring for some time. When spirits of chemical imbalance were commanded to leave, the two Christians felt a difference. At the next meeting, the mother reported her sweating had stopped. She was free of it.

A young mother didn't feel good about herself. As the bible group prayed, someone commanded a spirit of low-body self image to leave her. She broke into almost uncontrollable laughter. The spirit was gone. She was filled with joy.

Read on and rejoice in what the Lord is doing in these last days. Learn of victory after victory over spirit after spirit. Discover the awesome truth of the words of Jesus Christ, "The spirits are subject to you". (Luke 10:20) Know for a certainty that you have authority "over all the power of the enemy and nothing shall harm you". (Luke 10:19)

You're born again to win!

MOVING FORWARD

On the pages that follow, you can read about "great and mighty things which you do not know". (Jer. 33:6)

God, I believe, wants us to know of the great and mighty works He's performing today and would like to perform tomorrow - through you and I.

In the last days' global battle between God and Satan, we're on the winning side. Sickness and disease - all of it - is under our feet because we're in the body of Christ. And all of it is demonic. Every emotional, mental and physical sickness and pain is from the forces of the devil. No exceptions. The longer we minister, the more we're certain of that fact. You'll be reading of even Chemical and Hormonal Imbalance spirits cast out in the name of Jesus. Attention Deficit Disorder. Chronic Fatigue Syndrome. Tension and Stress. Onslaughts that come to "rob, kill and destroy". (John 10:10)

And consider this. Since all sickness is demonic and satanic spirits are involved, seldom can there be healing without deliverance. The causaative spirits must go! Whether the healing comes through the laying on of hands, anointing with oil, direct prayer, a prayer of agreement or a command in the name of Jesus, the spirit or spirits behind the problem will be ejected by the Holy Spirit. It simply figures. And it's all done in the name of Jesus, Who came to "set free". (Luke 4:18)

What a day to be alive! What a mighty God we serve! And what marvelous opportunities we have all around us to serve Him! So- let's start moving forward - to get free, set free and stay free. To bring freedom to the captives and glory to God!

Your Big Brother is a big winner

"When He (God) had disarmed the rulers and authorities, He made a public display of them, having triumphed over them through Him (Jesus)."(Co. 2:15)

Just call Him Jehovah Nissi, the Lord Your Victory, because that's what He is. And when you call on His name (the name of Jesus) you will be saved, according to Romans 4:13. And "sozo" the Greek word for "saved" includes deliverance and healing.

Philippians 2:10 states that at the name of Jesus every knee must bend in Heaven , on earth and under the earth. That about covers it, doesn't it?

What's more, this same Jesus has been given all authority in Heaven and on earth (where we are), according to Matthew 28:18. But since He doesn't need it on earth and we do, He delegates it to us, His believers. In Luke 10:19, the King of Kings declares, "I have given you authority to tread on serpents and scorpions (the devil and demons) and over all the power of the enemy and nothing shall hurt you". Quite a sweeping pronouncement.

Equally comprehensive is Jesus' promise from Matt. 16:19 and Matt. 18:18, "Whatever you shall bind on earth shall be bound in heaven, and whatever you shall loose on earth shall be loosed in heaven". "Bind" can also translate "refuse to permit" and "loose" can be translated "put off" or "cast out". That means you, fellow Christian, can refuse any physical, mental or emotional attack when it first begins. And - you can cast out the spirit any time after it has entered. Binding and loosing, Jesus calls them "the keys of the kingdom" (Matt. 16:19). As we use them, the gates of hell will not prevail against us (Matt 16:18).

Satan may "go about as a roaring lion" to devour us, as the apostle Peter writes (2 Peter 5:8), but when we resist him, he must flee from us. (James 4:7). And that goes for any of his cohorts.

Shucking off the spirits is so important that Jesus refers to it in his last statement in the gospel of Mark, "And these signs shall follow those who have believed: in My name they will cast out demons" (Mark 16:17). In Mark 16:20, we learn "the Lord worked with them and confirmed the word by the signs that followed". And He's still doing that today, confirming His words of the great commission. After all, we know from Hebrews 13:8 that Jesus Christ is the same yesterday, today and forever.

As you read on in this book, you'll see confirmation after confirmation, example after example of the Lord fulfilling His word, which endures forever (1 Peter 1:25). And you can better learn how to work with Him to deliver yourself and others.

The price of your victory

Let's look at the prepaid cost of our mental, physical and emotional health and healing - our deliverance from evil.

The price Jesus Christ paid is truly incomprehensible. In the 53rd Chapter of Isaiah, the prophet foresees, "Surely our sicknesses He Himself bore and our pains He carried," (Isaiah 53:4). And, "by His scourging we are healed". (Isaiah 53:5)

In the 52nd Chapter of Isaiah, we glimpse more of the Suffering Servant. "So His appearance was marred more than any man. And His form more than the sons of men." (Isaiah 52:14) Jesus looked as no man has ever looked. According to Isaiah 55:3, He was "like one from Whom men hid their face". They couldn't handle looking at Jesus. But we believers can begin to grasp the awful reality of the Lord's overwhelming suffering.

The Jewish Bible (Tanakh), (1985 edition), portrays even more graphically how horrible Jesus looked. And in this bible of unbelievers, you'll get a better idea of what the Romans did to His hands and feet. Just read Psalm 22. Every version of God's Word, of course, tells of the crown of thorns that dug into His head.

Why did the Son of God, God in the flesh, take on Himself every imaginable sickness and pain? So you and I wouldn't have to take it anymore! To tell the Lord you don't believe it's for today or that God doesn't want to heal everyone, (Matt. 8:17) says "He healed them all" to fulfill Isaiah 53), is almost like spitting in His face and turning away from His sacrifice. If you were Jesus, how would you feel after going through such tremendous torture only to have it rejected by someone you love?

By the substitutional victory of Jesus Christ over every evil that could plague us, we can walk victoriously, knowing the price has been paid to set us free.

Remember that Jesus Christ is the first-born among many brothers (and sisters). Our big brother won so that we can win in Him. Time after time, defeating all of our enemies. Psalm 118:10 says ("All nations (read 'demons') surround me (but) in the name of the Lord, I will surely cut them off." That's what this book is all about - cutting off our enemies. You'll read of Christians doing it, time after time.

Why not go and do likewise?

Your Father doesn't spare the horses

"But in all these things we overwhelmingly conquer through Him who loved us." (Rom. 8:37)

When our faith and actions are based on God's Word, we can expect results. That holds for healing and deliverance as well as any other area of living. To fight the good fight of faith, God has amply provided an abundance of scriptures to fortify ourselves with.

For example:

"I, the Lord, am your healer" (Ex. 15:26)
"I will remove sickness from your midst" (Ex. 23:25)
"I will fulfill the number of your days." (Ex. 23:26)
"And the Lord will remove from you all sickness" (Deut. 7:15)
"The Lord will cause your enemies who rise up against you to be defeated before you" (Deut. 28:7)
"They trusted, and Thou didst deliver them." (Ps. 22:14)
"Because he has loved Me, therefore I will deliver him" (Ps. 91: 14)
"Who heals all your diseases" (Ps.103:3)
"Bless the Lord, you His angels, mighty in strength, who obey the voice of His word!" (Ps. 103:20)
"He sent His word and healed them, and delivered them from their destructions." (Ps. 107:20)
"My son, give attention to My words; incline your ear to mysay ings. Do not let them depart from your sight; keep them in the midst of your heart. For they are life to those who find them, and health to all their body." (Prov. 4:20-22)
"No weapon that is formed against you shall prosper" (Is54:17)
"For I will restore you to health and I will heal you of your wounds" (Jer. 30:17)
"But for you who fear My name the sun of righteousness will rise with healing in its wings" (Mal. 4:12)
"And you will tread down the wicked, for they shall be ashes

under the soles of your feet" (Mal. 4:3)
"Behold, I have given you authority to tread upon serpents and scorpions, and over all the power of the enemy, and nothing shall injure you." (Luke 10:19)
"The spirits are subject to you" (Luke 10:20)
"And when evening had come, they brought to Him many who were demon possessed; and He cast out the spirits with a word, and healed all that were ill in order that what was spoken through Isaiah the prophet might be fulfillilled, saying "HE HIMSELF TOOK OUR INFIRMITIES AND CARRIED AWAY OUR DISEASES." (MATT. 8:17)
"Surely our sickness He Himself bore" (Is. 53:4)
"The chastening for our well-being fell upon Him, and by His scourging, we are healed. (Is. 53:5)
"for by His wounds you were healed." (I Peter 2:24)
"And Jesus was going about in all Galilee, teaching in their synagogues, and proclaiming the gospel of the kingdom, and healing every kind of sickness among the people." (Matt. 4:23)
"Truly, truly, I say to you, he who believes in Me, the works I do, he shall do also" (John 14:12)
"And whatever you ask (best translated "demand") in My name that will I do, that the Father may be glorifield in the Son." (John 14:13)
"I will give you the keys of the kingdom of heaven; and whatever you shall bind on earth shall be bound in heaven, and whatever you shall loose on earth shall be loosed in heaven." (Matt. 16:19)
"And these signs will accompany those who have believed; in My name they will cast out demons" (Mark 16:17)
"God seated Him (Jesus) at His right hand in the heavenly places, far above all rule and authority and power and dominion and every name that is named" (Eph. 1:20-21)
"and (God)raised us up with Him (Jesus) and seated us with Him, in the heavenly places, in Christ Jesus" (Eph:2:16)
"I pray that the eyes of your heart may be enlightened, so that you may know what is the surpassing greatness of His power toward us who believe." (I Cor. 1:18, 19)

The foregoing list is not, of course, complete. If you'd like to load up further with additional biblical ammunition, simply check a major concordance for words such as "heal", healing", "sickness", God's word, but strengthen your faith to start doing the works of Jesus. The possibilities are almost endless. The hurting people you can help will be almost legion. And your joy will be almost unspeakable!

A taste of deliverance from evil

"To set free those that are downtrodden".
(Luke 4:18)

One day, in the synagogue, Jesus read from Isaiah 61 and stated, in effect, that the Messiah had come. Later, in the gospel of Luke (10:21), we learn the Lord literally jumped for joy when He learned His disciples had successfully cast out demons in His name. And you can be sure He's still with us, rejoicing, as we too, drive out our spiritual enemies in His name through the Holy Spirit. That's still a vital part of His ministry, through us. It brings glory to the Father through the Son. (John 14:13)

So, rejoice, as we relate a few examples of Jesus setting the captives free today!

Ever had a nose that dripped like a worn-out faucet? My wife, Faye, did. And for three days she tried to turn off that faucet. Finally, two words came into her mind, "blossom spirit". Then she rebuked that spirit in the name of Jesus - and the dripping stopped in seconds. It was the same Holy Spirit Who raised Christ from the dead, living in her, Who told her the name of the enemy so she could cast it out in the name of Jesus.

We had just completed a telephone interview on a southern radio station. The show hostess, a Christian, gladly accepted prayer. And knowing that hard-working media mavens (and males) are often beset by spirits of tension and stress, we cast out those too-familiar spirits. The lady's happy comment was "It felt like a knot popped up from my stomach!" Our enemies would tie us in knots, but in the name of the Lord, we can cut them off. (Psalm 118:11)

Fred is a Christian who knows his rights. But until a momentous day in August of 1996, he hadn't exercised them very often. A couple of weeks earlier, Fred, in his seventies, had a physical attack that left him very weak and dizzy. After two weeks, half of his body had become numb.

At this point, Fred struck back. Out of his mouth came the words, "Oh, you spirit of numbness, I command you to leave me, in the name of Jesus Christ, the name above all names!" Sure enough, it happened and all of the numbness left Fred. He admitted he was surprised when he heard himself speaking that command. And he realizes the Holy Spirit in him helped with the outburst that ousted the demon.

Breast cancer is all too prevalent. No wonder Freda was concerned when a mammogram revealed she had a deep growth in one breast. The good news was that she was a very believing Christian and her very believing church rallied around her.

One evening, shortly after the ominous test results, four or five believers from her church gathered. Hands were laid on Freda and the spirit behind the growth was cast out in the name of the Lord.

Less than 72 hours later, Freda returned to the medical facility that had spotted the problem. New tests were taken. And the all-clear was sounded. No longer was there a sign of anything. Faith, the substance of things hoped for, the evidence of things unseen (Heb. 11:1 KJV) had provided the happy evidence.

A mighty Luis Palau crusade came to Chicago in the spring of 1996. One day, after many had come forward to receive Jesus Christ as Lord, a young Chriatian man wanted prayer. A Christian, helping at the meeting, offered to pray. The basic problem was depression, one of the devil's favorite advocates. The root problem was most likely rejection. (The young man was from a non-Christian country in the Mideast.)

The brief, but effective, deliverance began with the departure of spirits of tension and stress. Anxiety followed. Then fear left. Finally rejection and the fear of it left. Of course, the spirit of depression itself had to go - and the young man was set free - after years of demonic oppression.

Another young man, after the same meeting, was ready for prayer. His was a physical problem, what seemed to be bronchitis with a cough involved. But, physical healing is just as easy for Jesus as emotional healing. When spirits of sinusitis, allergic rhinitis and catarrh were cast out, this young man, an assistant pastor, also felt better., In fact, he was so pleased with the results that he kept commenting about how well he felt!

God is moving to take back the media. And that includes the ever-present telephone. Pastor John McCall of Baltimore Christian Faith Center speaks at meetings around the country. Once, some time after he'd taught at a church in Kansas, a lady from there called him in Baltimore. She was desperate. Terminal bone cancer had her on crutches - and on the ropes. Braces on both legs protected the fragile bones. But nothing is impossible with God, and Pastor McCall knew it. He took authority in the name of Jesus Christ. He cast out and cursed the cancer.

What happened was mind-boggling - and faith-building. Instantly, the power of God came on the lady and all pain left her. Shortly afterward, she returned to the hospital for a check-up. The findings? This once-cancer victim was totally healed. No more braces, no more crutches. No more eroding bones. And she went back to work - home free through the implementation of God's health care plan.

Ardis had a hearing problem that began in her mouth. No, we're not kidding. She had a severely abscessed tooth that was pulled. This led to temporary loss of hearing. After she could hear again, there remained an echo in her ears. Not a pleasant curcumstance.

At this point, a praying Christian received a word of knowledge from God. Ardis had a spirit of distortion. When that was cast out, she turned her head from side and discovered there was no more echo.

Jesus Christ took all of our sicknesses and pains. Not even an echo should remain!

A family in our church decided to take the kids and enjoy a nice dinner. They were hungry and the restuarant seemed inviting. However, they were in for some surprises. Not in the culinary department, either.

After all four in the family began to eat, demonic attacks set in on all of them.

Mom began to feel sandpaper-like roughness in her throat. Even when she rebuked, the feeling moved around in her throat. Dad got a headache. The children picked up stomach discomfort. Yet, the food tasted fine.

What was the problem? There could have been satanic activity throughout the restaurant. More likely, this attack was aimed at the members of the family - all beginning to move strongly for God. The devil hates that.

As we prayed for the parents in church, the throat problem and headache seemed to be gone. Nevertheless, we prayed against residence spirits - and there was no reaction.

Then, also with hands on, we prayed for dad against a head-blocking spirit - and he felt the power of God. Commanding prayer, plus hands-on from dad, brought a strong presence of the Holy Spirit on mom, who began to reel back under the freeing power of God. In this case, we commanded a throat-blocking spirit to leave, also in Jesus' name.

Please, don't be be afraid to eat in restaurants. This was an unusual situation. This may have been solely an attack on the members of this godly family. It may not have happened to any of the other diners. Satan is trying to pick-off Christians. But these Christians have authority over him in the name of Jesus Christ! He told us, in John 8:31, if we continue in His word we would indeed be his disciples and we would know the truth and that truth would set us free. If we focus the light, it will overcome the darkness!

More encouraging developments occurred in a couple of nursing homes recently. In the first case, I was talking to a lady who was hard-of-hearing. She wasn't following the conversation. But, as I was speaking, in my mind I rebuked a deaf spirit - and she began to hear.

The second experience was in another nursing home. This lady wasn't responding to the sinners prayer. Noticing a Catholic magazine for the deaf, I took authority over a deaf spirit, in my mind as I was speaking. She began to move her lips and became a born-again Christian. Point: yes, you can take authority over evil spirits by speaking to them in your mind.,

Perhaps in your city, there's an annual Taste of____________, where would-be buyers can sample restaurant goodies. What you've just read should provide a taste of what Jesus Christ is doing through His believing vessels. The Great Shepherd has set a table beforeus in the midst of our enemies (Ps. 23:5). Taste on and see that the Lord is good ! (Ps. 118:1) Then enter into His good provision!

Surefire winners in spiritual warfare

"For the weapons of our warfare are not of the flesh, but divinely powerful for the destruction of fortresses." (II Cor. 10:4)

Spiritual warfare! There's a descriptive phrase totally unknown to the non-Christian world. But most Christians are aware of it. Not surprising, for Christians are the devil's primary targets. He already has the others in his kingdom, although they don't know it.

Unfortunately, most Christians are uncomfortable with that term. They'd rather the devil would go away so they wouldn't have to fight. Equally, unfortunately, that won't happen. The apostle Peter warns in I Peter 5:8 that our enemy, the devil, prowls about like a roaring lion, seeking someone to devour." Peter also follows with the prescribed response to enemy attacks, "but resist him, firm in your faith". James adds (James. 4:7) "resist the devil and he will flee from you".

So we shouldn't be scaredy cats, but confident Christians, firm in our faith. Remember the words of God in Isaiah 41:10, "Do not fear, for I am with you", and He is El Shaddei, the God Who is more than enough. And to fend off and drive out the mental, emotional and physical incursions of the enemy, He has given us more than enough weapons to win every time.

THE NAME OF JESUS

First and foremost is the mighty name of Jesus Christ, in Whom we live and move and have our being. (Acts 17:28) From Philippians 2:9, we know that "God has bestowed on Him the name which is above every name". Why? "That AT THE NAME OF JESUS, EVERY KNEE SHOULD BOW".

And we have the use of His name! In fact, a sign that should follow every believer (Mark 16:7) is “in My name, they will cast out demons.” Prov. 18:10 states, “The name of the Lord is a strong tower, the righteous runs into it and is safe.” (And remember, Romans 5:17 says you have received the gift of righteousness and are to “reign in life through the one, Christ Jesus”).

Don’t forget, either, that in John 14:13, Jesus promises that whatever we demand (best translation from the Greek) in His name He will do “that the Father may be glorified in the Son.”

He did exactly that in a nursing home where a lady complained of a painful foot. When we commanded the spirit of pain to leave, the lady said, “when you said ‘Jesus’ it was like a zap hit my foot.” and the pain left entirely. In that same nursing home, a deaf young lady who could barely speak, commanded the deaf spirit to leave her in the name of Jesus and the broad smile that followed attested to the immediate sign of better hearing. Whether you drive out a spirit from yourself or from someone else, remember, Jesus, by the power of the Holy Spirit, is doing it for you.

The world too often swears with that name, but we Christians should always swear by it - and use it! I believe the all-powerful name of Jesus Christ is the number one weapon of our warfare.

All of the above is based on and according to the Bible, the word of God. Jesus lets us know in John 17:17 that God’s word is truth (reality). That’s from the same high-priestly prayer in which the Lord asks the Father to keep us safe from the evil one by the power “of the name you gave Me.” (John 17:11 & 15 NIV)

THE WORD OF GOD

God’s word, in our hearts and on our lips, is a tremendous

weapon. In Romans 10:9, we learn the principle that as we believe in our hearts and confess or speak with our mouths, we will be saved (and the Greek word for 'saved' includes 'delivered'). Very often, Faye and I will speak appropriate scripture(s) as we bind or loose in the name of Jesus.

When you speak God's word you (1) bring angels on the scene to perform it (Psalm 103:20), (2) you, like Jesus in Matt.4, remind the devil of the scriptural reality and assurance of the legality of what you're doing, (3) building your own faith, which comes "with hearing " the word of God" (Rom. 8:17 KJV). Also, you are showing faith and expecting God to reward you (Heb. 11:6) and that pleases Him.

Additionally, after deliverance, it's wise to renew your mind by God's word (Rom. 12:12). This will build you up, and change attitudes that could have necessitated your deliverance. Knowing and using God's word will help you stay free!

The following awesome example of the power of God's word is chronicled in our book, "God's Health Care Plan".

After a desperate mother commanded a new brain into her brain-atrophied, epileptic, retarded three-year-old son, she my wife and I, thanked God as we spoke and claimed over and over (for at least 15 minutes) Psalm 23:3 that God restored the boy's soul (mind, emotions and will) and given him "a sound mind" (II Tim. 1:7 (KJV). As the mother drove her son home to Iowa, she kept confessing those scriptures and thanking God they had come to pass. Less than two days later, they did come to pass. The child developed a new curiosity and even his skeptical father noticed a change in the shape of his son's head. Later testing showed there indeed was a new brain. The neurologist said of the once hopeless situation, "the sky's the limit."

SPIRITUAL GIFTS

A third weapon of our warfare is God's provision of the

Gifts of the Spirit (I Cor. 12 & 14). These supernatural endowments can bring very helpful manifestations. The Word of Knowledge and Discerning of Spirits are two ways God provides important information we otherwise wouldn't be aware of. These gifts can are among the a-bombs of spiritual warfare.

A man at one of our home bible fellowships was finally freed from pain when the Lord gave a member of the group the words 'lumbago'. When that spirit was addrressed, the man was set free. While we were praying for (and delivering) someone in the back of the church, the Lord indicated one of his problems was a spirit. He noticed a definite release after we cast it out. He also admitted this spirit of poverty had formed an outlook and expectation. The spirit, which ran in the family , was an inherited spirit. In the chapter that follows, you'll learn more about the Word of Knowledge.

PRAISE

A fourth weapon God gives His people is praise. Paul and Silas sang praises to God while they were shackled in prison - and He sent a minor earthquake to break their chains. (Acts 16:25, 26). Praise can break chains today and remove demonic yokes. Faye often gets free from physical ailments as she sings praise to God. Psalm 106:47 (KJV) tells us to "give thanks unto Thy holy name, and to triumph in Thy praise". Praising God can magnify Him (in our own minds), also bring His even greater presence, and give us more confidence as we battle the enemy. On one occasion when I praised God with a painful shoulder. I was so high on the Lord that all the pain left quickly with one rebuke in the name of Jesus.

Praising God after He's delivered us from something builds faith to refuse to speak negative words on the subject that could help us lose our healing...such as "I didn't think it could last", "I'm starting to hurt again", etc. Instead praise can help us confidently help us to trust God as we refuse any old or new symptoms in His Son's name. It affects our attitude and expectation and let's the Lord pour in more power. Remember how David encouraged himself in the Lord? You can do it, too!

PRAYING IN THE SPIRIT

When we don't know how to pray as we should, we can pray in the spirit (in tongues)(Rom: 8:25). Often, in deliverance, we can't determine what spirit to speak to next. Perhaps the physical healing, if this is needed, still hasn't manifested. Maybe there's some kind of blockage or a root spirit that must be evicted. At this point, when we specifically pray in the spirit, the Lord may provide a word of knowledge. The Holy Spirit is our helper (one of His seven names in the Greek). Often, we'll do this in even one-on-one ministry, or I may do it praying for myself. In our home bible group, all of us may pray in tongues and the Lord may give someone a word or an approach to take.

For example, one night, a lady in the group had a vision showing a particular demon spirit. We were then able to proceed through driving out a blocking spirit.

When we pray inthe spirit, the Spirit Himself intercedes for us (Rom. 8:25) and prays the perfect prayer, or says the perfect words to God the Father. Unbeatable!

THE BLOOD OF JESUS

Our sixth weapon is what paid for Jesus' atonement that made all of this possible. As we realize the price He paid, we can feel more confident of moving in the victory the atonement of Jesus has provided. The blood of Jesus, poured out of His body and on to the Heavenly mercy seat of God undergirds us and constantly reminds our Father of His Son's sacrifice for us. It also reminds Satan and his clan of their defeat.

I recall once starting to move to my desk to note Christian information about the blood. Suddenly, I became dizzy and could scarcely reach the desk. Never have I had that problem since.

Faye and I usually bind the devil and cover ourselves with the blood of Jesus when doing deliverance.

To sum up, as you refuse or cast out spirits in the name of Jesus, don't hesitate to speak the appropriate scripture(s), be open to the Holy Spirit for words of knowledge, praise the Lord Who's doing the work, and remember, it's all possible because of the blood sacrifice of Jesus Christ. Through Him, God has given us everything we need for life and holiness (II Peter 1:3)!

God would reveal the enemy

"Now concerning spiritual gifts, brethren, I do not want you to be unaware" (I Cor. 12:1)

When it comes to driving out spirits, the Lord doesn't leave us orphans. Often, as we minister, He provides information that helps show us which mountain to speak to. He, of course, will do the same for all His people. There's work to be done, and the Holy is designated to be our helper. And words of knowledge (one of the nine Gifts of the Spirit) He provides are key to handling particular problems.

One example occurred in an extraordinary case. Fran called complaining of multiple problems. First, she had a throbbing headache so severe she could hardly hold her head up. Second, the atmosphere in the house she rented was heavy and strange. One night, a lady friend sleeping in one of the bedrooms, reported a hand touching her during the night. And, over a period of time, Fran and her daughter would put objects in one room and find them in another. Uncomfortable, she prepared to move.

Her landlord happened to be a mortician who had lived in the house. As I quietly prayed inthe spirit, a word like "disjointment" came into my mind. Fran went on to mention that the undertaker was suspected by neighbors of performing autopsies in the basement. Then, "disjointment " made sense.

In the name of Jesus, I commanded a residual spirit of disjointment to leave. The results were startling. On the phone, Fran reported the heaviness and oppressions in the room had lifted. She said, "the air seems clean". Then she added, "the headache is gone!"

The Lord had wanted to bring light into darkness. So, through one word of knowledge, He cleaned up the environment and cleared out the headache. Both problems had been caused by that same spirit. To complete the picture, a few weeks later Fran told us that objects were no longer moving from one room to another. God had done a thorough work!

Gloria, a young wife, had been hoping for years to become pregnant. Nothing seemed to help. As she was receiving prayer, one of the ladies in the bible study received a word of knowledge. And she spoke the words "thyroid-stimulating hormone deficiency'. Amazed, Gloria told the group these were the exact words of diagnosis spoken to her by a physician.

When a spirit of thyroid stimulating hormone deficiency was cast out in the name of Jesus, Gloria burst into uncontrollable laughter. She laughed and laughed and laughed and had trouble stopping.

Will she become pregnant? I don't know. But we do know that God had provided surprising information and then filled His daughter with his joy. Is that scriptural? In Psalm 126, you can read, "When the Lord brought back the captive ones of Zion, we were like those who dream. Then our mouth was filled with laughter."

It was time for prayer at a home meeting. Joan suffered pain in her chest, lungs, sides and hips. When we commanded it to leave, it didn't. Shortly afterward, while we prayed, I felt the Lord was telling me to ask if anyone had experienced sadness at at the age of eight or nine. Was it the Holy Spirit or my own thought?

Finally, I did ask the question. Good thing. Joan told us, through tears, that when she was eight, both her father and her brother had died. It had been a traumatic year. Now an adult, Joan forgave God and others she, from childhood, held anger and bitterness toward. She was set free from scarcely remembered but deeply entrenched spiritual and emotional hurts.

The door had opened to heal the physical pain. As my wife laid hands on Joan's chest, we prayed for healing in Jesus' name. Joan reported the heat traveled from the hand throughout the entire painful body areas. Our God is a loving, compassionate and healing Father.

A major Christian ministry had just completed a series of meetings in a Southern city. Several attendees remained in the auditoriun. A group of people gathered around as lady in a wheel chair. They were praying for her. Another Christian was watching. As she was praying in the spirit, she felt a pain in her neck. She could scarcely move her neck.

With that aching neck, this lady walked to the one in the wheel chair. She told her, and those in the group, about the neck pain she was experiencing. It happened that the lady in the wheel chair did indeed have a large knot in her neck. Realizing she had heard from God, the Christian who had just felt the pain, laid hands on the one in the wheel chair and said "come out of her in the name of Jesus!" Almost immediately, the knot in the neck disappeared.

Why did the Lord give that word of knowledge for the healing of the neck but nothing for the damaged body? Perhaps the neck healing would build the lady's faith for a healing that would get her on her feet.

As we walked down the hall of a nursing home, one of the aides approached us. She remembered us from the bible study. She had this to relate: she had recently returned from Philadelphia. While she was there, she went with a relative to a small Christian church. At that church, a woman approached her and told her of a sickness the first lady had, but which couldn't be determined by her appearance. God had, of course, given the second lady a word of knowledge. Armed with that information, she prayed and God healed the visitor from Chicago. There was amazement and awe in her voice as she related her miracle. Truly, our God is an awesome God!

When do you get a word from God and how does it manifest? You get it when He wills to give it to you. (1 Cor. 12) Whom might He use? Any born-again Christian available at the time. Manifestation can come in any of a number of ways. It could be a thought dropped into your mind from out of the blue. It could be a knowing inside. It could be a vision, open or otherwise. Perhaps a dream. It might be a feeling of pain in the area someone is suffering. You may feel a lightness or unction in your spirit (located in your belly) when something is mentioned or you ask the Lord for help. It may be a leading in a particular direction.

One such word I'll never forget came while I was praying in the spirit before a home bible fellowship meeting. I saw dimly, but surely, a thumb with a split thumbnail.

During the meeting, almost apologetically, I asked if anyone had a finger problem. One middle-aged lady stated she had a thumb with a split nail. When we prayed, God took away the pain and subsequently healed her.

But there's more to the story. The lady we'll call Audrey, had told no one, not even her husband (who was at the meeting) of her problem. Her loving Father, she realized was the only Person who knew. And He cared enough to tell and then heal.

This was very important to Audrey. She had been put down in life often. Her own father had stood by again and again when her mother would hang her by the hands (when she was a teenager). She had no positive father image. Consequently, it had been difficult for Audrey to look at God as a loving Father. Now she knew He was just that. She said later that when she was tempted to doubt that her Heavenly Father really loves her, she remembers the split thumbnail. One divine word of knowledge can change someone's life!

It was night in the brightly lighted area between buildings of a large prison complex. As a ministering team was walking through to go on home, a police officer approached and wanted help for an inmate and his wife. The inmate's father had been killed in a highway accident. The daughter-in-law knew. The son didn't. One member of the team would tell the man of his father's sudden death. With the help of the Lord, he did - and provided what comfort he could.

In the waiting room, his wife was nervous and praying. (Both she and her husband were Christians.) She asked the church group for prayer. Through a word of knowledge, one member of the team felt the lady had a stomach problem. He asked - and yes, she had ulcers. When that spirit was expelled in the name of Jesus, her stomach pain left with it. Yet, it also happened she had overall body pain. When arthritis was kicked out, she felt much better. Now, she could more easily cope with the sudden and shocking death of her father-in-law and be an even stronger support for her husband. The word of knowledge - more proof the Lord is with us in times of need!

It was a bible study and prayer meeting. At the time of prayer, one of the attenders said the Lord had impressed something on him before the meeting. Someone there had a problem sleeping. Did anyone there have such a problem? No one responded. Well, sometimes what seems like a word of knowledge will prove otherwise.

But, a mother at the meeting remembered that her son, Kenny, could be the one. He had swollen and enlarged adenoids. And the boy was there at the time. So, hands were laid on him and the adenoid infirmity spirit was cast out in the name of Jesus. He noticed a difference immediately. More importantly, he began sleeping better that very night!

Mom and dad, knowing their authority in Jesus have been keeping that spirit off of their son. So, he continues to sleep much better.

God's precious words of knowledge - through any of His people to help any people!

The avoidance of slavery to sin

"You shall have no other gods before (besides) Me." (Exodus 20:23)

Before we get into the substance of this chapter, we should make this preliminary comment. Sickness, or any kind of affliction doesn't necessarily come about because we've sinned. The devil doesn't have to have an opening, just our permission. And we give that automatically if we don't refuse the attack. James 4:7 always applies. It's up to us to resist in the name of Jesus. But, when we are in unconfessed sin, we're out from God's protective umbrella and in the devil's territory. That's a dangerous place to be.

To God, known sin is no slight matter. It's turning away from Him, the one who loves us with an everlasting love. With sin, we're putting the god of this world above our Almighty Father.

That's why God considers sin idolatry.

Chapter and verse? There's a big clue in Ezekial 8:3, where the Holy Spirit showed the prophet the inner court of the temple in Jerusalem, "where the seat of the idol of jealousy, which provokes to jealousy, was located." Right inside God's own temple! That's where His priests had set up that idol! Now there's a slap in the face!

In Ezekial 8:10, we discover about "all the idols of the house of Israel" in the court of the temple. More than one idol. That's even worse.

But, before we condemn them, let's look at ourselves. We, too, are priests to God (1 Peter 2:9) and each Christian is a temple of the Holy Spirit. (1 Cor. 3:16) Do we build and/or bow to idols of fear, greed, self-pity, pride, resentment, etc? Actually, anything or anyone we put on a par with God is idolatry.

While we're on this perhaps uncomfortable subject , which I didn't originally plan to explore, we should realize that many items we may not have considered sin God considers sin. The truth is, anything which is contrary to the word of God is sin. "Whatever is not from faith is sin." (Rom. 14:23)

For example, since God's word tells us hundreds of times not to fear, fear is a sin. It may be the most prevalent sin in today's scared-silly, bad-news-press society. And fear is a great door-opener to other emotional as well as physical spirits. By itself, it's dangerous bondage that keeps us, among other things, from witnessing and making intelligent and Godly decisions.

Consider anxiety. Jesus tells us not to be anxious. (Luke 12:22 and elsewhere) He also commands us not to worry . (John 14:27)

Stress and tension? "Let not your heart not be troubled. (also John 14:27)

Then there's that negative robber, doubt. "Without faith, it's impossible to please him." (Heb. 11:6) James 1:6,7 reminds us the double-minded person shouldn't expect to receive anything from God.

When we're in bondage to sin, we become slaves to it, which keeps us from being the best bond-slaves of Jesus Christ. And, God says, (Ex. 20:5), "You shall not worship or serve them; for I, the Lord your God am a jealous God".

Awareness of the idolatry of sin should give us new resolve to resist the spirits that attack us, confess when we yield, (1 John 1:8), and live under the shelter of the Most High. When we come clean, it's easier to clean up on the devil!

The due process of elimination

"In the name of the Lord, I will surely cut them off." (Psalm 118:10)

Why don't some people get healed? The answers are manifold: lack of knowledge, incorrect teaching, wanting to stay sick, unbelief, unforgiveness. (It's never God's fault. Matt. 8:17 states Jesus healed them all, to fulfill Isaiah 53 that He bore our sickness and pains)

PLUS - and we believe this is very major - physical healing is often blocked by emotional spirits. These spirits may be the entire cause of the physical problem. Or, they may have opened the door to the physical infirmity and are holding it in place. In either scenario, they must be dealt with.

Headaches are common, but their causes will vary. Marie had migraines, those knife-like intruders that can cut into our well being.

When Marie wanted prayer, we told that migraine spirit to leave. But it didn't. She had no relief. Brief conversation indicated she was in stress and also holding anger and resentment toward someone close to her. (Remember that song, "You Always Hurt the One You Love"?) Knowing this, we cast out, in order, spirits of stress, anger and resentment. Marie noticed the difference.Then, we commanded spirits of migraine to leave and they did. Through the name of Jesus those headaches were behind her. But for that to happen, three other enemies had to be cut off. Several years later, Marie recalled what God had done for her and remarked on how well she'd been feeling!

Here's a case of the entire head pain caused by other spirits. Leslie had an extremely severe headache. Her face confirmed the intense pain. "I can't stand it", she said. She was down into understandable doldrums. But at the name of

Jesus, every knee shall bend. And, in this situation, there were quite a few.

First, we cast out discouragement, followed by chemical imbalance. Obsequiesness came next. Since there had been past occult involvement, Faye and I drove out inherited witchcraft, divination, astrology, black and white magic and ouija. A generational curse was also broken. Leslie was beginning to feel relief.

Then came anxiety, inflammation, arthritis, dizziness (she told us this sometimes occurred). She had a history of very high blood pressure from time to time, so we commanded a spirit of blood pressure imbalance to leave. Finally, swelling and inflammation were cast out.

Now, Leslie reported, the headache was completely gone. Link by link, the chain had been broken. Thanks be to God Who gives us the victory through our Lord Jesus Christ! (1 Cor. 15:57)

Here's a somewhat similar situation. Clarice had been stung by a yellowjacket a few days earlier. The pain, though, was still around. It had moved from the neck to the shoulder and to the upper back. Although she had been rebuking the back pain, Clarice's hurt still existed.

In our commanding prayer, we tried the obvious. Any poison was rebuked. Pain, inflammation and soreness were also spoken to in Jesus name. All to no avail. Then came these emotional spirits: fear, anxiety , tension and stress. Clarice felt peace, but she still felt pain. Finally, praying in the spirit brought rejection to mind. So we commanded spirits of rejecation, self-rejection and fear of rejection to leave. Clarice swung her head, neck and upper body around a few times. The pain had gone. Those rejection spirits had kept it on her.

And what about the not-so-yellowjacket that had stung her? Most likely, that sting had brought the initial pain, but the rejection spirits had allowed it to stay and move around her body. Frankly, we don't know. We do know that emotional and physical enemies left Clarice. And the entire deliverance took around five minutes.

Carl had a history of panic attacks. He also suffered from high blood pressure. An appointment at Mayo Clinic was on the calendar.

Happily, Carl was very open to prayer during our phone conversation. And the Holy Spirit began to move. In this order, the following emotional spirits were cast: stress and tension, anxiety, panic attack, fear of rejection and self-rejection. At this point, I went for the physical spirits and cast out a spirit of high blood pressure and then blood presssure imbalance. Throughout the freeing process, Carl was feeling better and better.

Some weeks later, I spoke with Carl again. He shared his good news. He had kept the appointment at Mayo Clinic - and received "a clean bill of health"! So often, when the emotional spirits go, the physical follow after.

Abortion

Abortion invariably seems to cause long-lasting emotional anguish. This is common knowledge. But the suffering doesn't have to continue. Before-and-after-the-fact spirits can be dislodged in the name of Jesus. Otherwise such emotional spirits can prevent healing.

Winnie had a prolapsed uterus. Prayer against this proved of little effect, until the following spirits were cast out: anxiety, inherited fear and depression. Then we learned about the abortion, long ago, before she had become a Christian. When we addressed a spirit of abortion in the name of Jesus, there was no release. However, when we commanded a spirit of guilt and then shame to leave Winnie, she experienced a definite release. The same effect came when a spirit of murder was ejected. In this case, there was no spirit of abortion abiding in her. But causative and post-abortion spirits were the deep enemies.

Now, we went on to speak to physical problem spirits. When we commanded what we call the sinus chain (which includes sinusitis, allergic rhinitis, catarrh, post-nasal drip and bronchitis), Winnie's nasal passages seemed to open and there was flowing in this area. We prayed against a spirit of exzcema (which had been in her fingers for three years) and blood rushed to her hands.

Finally, we again prayed against the prolapsed uterus - and Winnie felt a new freedom in that area. This hadn't occurred earlier. Obviously, emotional spirits were blocking physical healing. Now, Winnie was feeling better, emotionally and physically. How long did it take? At most, a half hour. And, of course, Faye equipped Winnie with the list of spirits so she could stand against attempts to return.

Salvation blockage

This one is so important, we're headlining it.

So many of us are believing God for the salvation of family and friends. We want them in the kingdom of God, not on the highway to hell.

El and Audrey Swanson had a former neighbor who had moved to the Southwest. He was terminally ill of cancer. He did not know Jesus Christ as Lord.

Christians in this man's new location were witnessing to him about Jesus Christ. But, he just didn't seem to be able to ask Jesus into his heart.

One day, as El and Audrey were praying, God dropped the answer into El's mind. The blocker was a spirit of rejection of receiving Jesus.

The Swansons called long distance. Their friend was sleeping, so they left a message. After he awoke, he returned the call. On the phone, in a matter of minutes, he prayed and received Jesus Christ as Lord and Savior. Weeks later he died. Today he's in Heaven - because the Swansons prayed and God answered through a word of knowledge. And also because El Swanson cast out that spirit that blocked the reception of Jesus.

Is someone you know on the brink of salvation but seemingly unable to make the move? Consider the possibility of demonic blockage by a spirit of rejection of receiving Jesus. If that isn't it, ask the Lord. He wants that person in His family even more than you do. He understands the horror of the alternative.

Marriage Blockers

The devil hates God's institutions. He works hard to destroy them, especially marriage. Look at the divorce statistics. They're readily available. But more difficult is discovering the number of unhappy or not-so-solid marriages.

Helen's marriage was shaky. A Christian, and a midwesterner, she believed in family values. Her husband and children were very important to her. She loved them.

But she needed outside help. A deliverance session brought just that. Jesus saves - people, psyches and marriages.

First, stress and tension were addressed and Helen was smiling. The list of spirits that followed is long, but we think you should be aware of it. The fear and rejection group included fear, anxiety, inherited rejection, inherited fear, residual fear, self rejection, inadequacy and fear of it. Inherited rage, inherite anger and hostility were then cast out. Unworthiness, depression, discouragement and low body self image were loosed. Helen was getting releases down the line - and knew it.

Resentment, a root of bitterness, rebellion, perverse spirit, chemical, metabolic and thyroid imbalance were driven off. Inherited poverty and inherited lack and frugality were next. When love of money left, Helen yawned. Sadness was dispatched. Then residual doubt with a big yawn - a strong blocker.

Physical healing followed. Pain left with inherited arthritis. The pain in her joints and pressure on the balls of her feet took off when a spirit of bursitis did. Inflammation (often combining with pain) was cast out. Now inherited sinusitis, rhinitis and catarrh were addressed. And Helen felt lighter. Finally a spirit of vanity was loosed - along with a deep yawn.

The cleansing was completed. Note the many inherited spirits that barnacled Helen. And know the marriage is now better. God is still in the restoring business!

Bonita had problems. She was hurting, primarily emotionally. Physically, she had an undiagnosed hard substance in her stomach area. Also she was considerably overweight. Not healthy. Emotionally, she had suffered death in the family and rejection from a friend.

The Lord delivered her in this order: rejection, fear of rejection, depression and fear of depression (problems here since she was sixteen), discouragement. When she was a child , she heard her mother tell her dad she was going leave. Mom was kidding, but little Bonita didn't know that. A spirit of abandonment was cast out. The came self-condemnation and self-pity, Because she was overweight, she had a low-body self-image.This spirit was also ejected in the name of Jesus. At this point, she felt like laughing, often a reaction when low-body self-image leaves.

Then authority was taken over a spirit of obesity and one of hernia. With the latter, Bonita felt something move in the middle of her body. The noticeable end result of the session was great peace for Bonita. Emotionally, she had been healed, and probably physically as well.

Luella was at a business meeting when she experienced shortage of breath. For some years, she had an enlarging heart and hypertension of the lungs - plus severe rheumatoid arthritis. And she was told she could use heart and lung transplants. At the time of her phone call, she had taken leave from work. She was in no condition to continue with interstate travel since that breath occurrence (in 1995). Luella had called for much-needed help.

Commanding prayer began with the expulsion of stress and tension. Then anxiety and fear left. Rejection, fear of rejection and self-rejection followed.

Now we addressed the physical demons. Luella felt better when a spirit of rheumatoid arthritis was cast out in the name of Jesus. Bursitis and inflammation were ejected - and she could lift her leg higher. Pain left and Luella's hands felt better. After sciatica took off, she could rotate her shoulder without cracking. Stiffness was cast out bringing more improvement. When we spoke to a spirit of hypertension of the lungs, she breathed more freely. After residual stiffness left, her knees felt fine. Residual arthritis departed and Luella's hands could nearly close. Thyroid and hormonal imbalance were ejected and her breathing improved even more. Now, Luella could more freely move her arms, shoulders and hands.

All of the above took about thirty minutes. Years of hurt were handled quickly - through the use of our rod of authority, the mighty name of our mighty Lord, Jesus Christ!

Carrie called from the Caribbean. She had been reading "God's Health Care Plan". She needed prayer. In depression, dizzy and off-balance, with an ear infection, epileptic seizures and memory loss, Carrie was devilishly afflicted - and still in her thirties.

When we cast out trauma, Carie said it left as soon as we spoke in the name of Jesus. Next to leave was bio-chemical imbalance. She also felt release on epilepsy and a major reaction when depression was uprooted. Deliverance continued with pharmakia (drugs) and inherited occult spirits. Fear, dizziness, anxiety, stress and tension were cast from her. When we spoke to a spirit of ear infection, her ear pain left. Discovering Carrie had been rejected at home and at school, we cast out inherited rejection.

The discernible end result was that Carrie felt "much better" and experienced a new peace.

Î should add, that during deliverance, we often may speak to spirits that aren't there. But, the best way is to cover the waterfront and if sometimes you come up dry, nothing is lost!

Rose was a conscientious worker. Yet, for too long, she had to take off and spend much of her time in bed.

What was going on? Dizziness, blurred vision. Her arms and legs seemed weak. Her doctor's diagnosis: myasthenia gravis, "brought on by stress". Rose was an executive and a busy one. Stress had moved in.

In twelve minutes, Jesus made a tremendous difference. He delivered Rose from a host of spirits...starting with stress, tension, anxiety and fear. Then came three imbalance spirits: chemical, biochemical, and hormonal, followed by low body self image. Now - dizziness...depression and discouragement, the rejection and inadequacy spirits. Then anger, wrath and resentment were cast out. At this point, Rose forgave one or more people. Next, she lost chronic fatigue syndrome, narcolepsy - and finally - myasthenia gravis.

After all of the above - Rose's vision was no longer blurred. Her dizziness was nearly gone and she reported feeling "good". Her morale as well as her body was much improved!

Marvin had been in a church that didn't believe in divine healing. It had, in fact, forced a pastor to leave who did believe God heals today. So where was Marvin to go for help? He had heard of us through "God's Health Care Plan" and he called.

Physically, Marvin was bothered with itching in his genital area. After talking with him and learning he had been in the occult before he became a Christian, we cast out a spirit of sorcery. He felt a crawling feeling. Then, in Jesus name, we spoke again, this time, I believe, against a residual spirit of sorcery, that crawling feeling stopped - the spirit had left.

When an inherited spirit of hormonal imbalance was driven out, Marvin felt a coolness in his body. His siblings had opposed his marriage; he had been the major family wage-earner. So we cast out wrath and rage. Marvin also had difficulty concentrating - and was then delivered from a spirit of attention deficit disorder.

Now we commanded a spirit of genital infirmity to leave. Marvin felt tingling in his scrotum. And - the itching was gone. Jesus Christ had delivered him emotionally and physically.

Little things can mean a lot. Recently, after a certain amount of computer software frustration, I began to feel quite tired. That's uncommon for me. And I made two mistakes. I spoke about being very tired and I didn't think of spirits that might have gotten on me.

As I started taking a nap at 5 PM, I decided to command depression to leave me. I felt better. Self-pity and discouragement and one or two others were addressed. There was improvement. The expulsion of spirits had made a difference.

Depression has almost never been a problem during my many years as a Christian. From the above incident, I can realize first hand how it can affect someone without that person realizing what was happening. Just one more proof that emotional spirits can cause physical problems. At the first sign of a downturn of any kind, we should rebuke obvious causes, or ask the Lord what to take authority over.

Is depression a major and prevalent enemy? AMI, the Alliance for the Mentally Ill states that crippling depression strikes over 11 million Americans each year.

Sam is a farmer who loves Jesus. He also cares for his wife and child. But there have been problems with the girl, including getting her out of bed in the morning. We suggested that fear, abandonment and fear of abandonment could be attacking the child before she goes to school. Those spirits, like any others, can be bound.

Sam himself indicated a couple of inherited spirits that were bugging him. The first was anger that passed down the family line. When we cast out that spirit in Jesus' name, he felt a release. The second inherited spirit was lust. It may have entered with Playboy magazines brought into the family home by someone during Sam's youth.

When we drove out an inherited spirit of lust, Sam said "yeah!" and felt a pronounced tingle all over him. God had set him free from two major enemies.

The Lord likes to direct His people, too. Sam wanted to be planted as a Christian light in the world. When we prayed, the power of God came on him strongly. It was a manifestation that God heard, wanted what Sam did, and would move for him.

Being a Christian can be a very exciting and satisfying life!

Freedom brings blessings

"And whenever you stand praying, forgive, if you have anything against anyone; so that your Father also who is in heaven may forgive you your transgressions." (Mark 11:25)

The sweet little lady in the nursing home was hurting. She was experiencing sharp pain. Faye and I commanded the spirit of pain to leave her, but it stayed. Why? Because there was someone that nice lady was holding a grudge against - and that was holding her healing back.

When she agreed to forgive and did it, when she asked God to forgive her for being unforgiving, then we spoke against that spirit of pain in the name of Jesus Christ - and the pain left.

You never know. So many people stuff resentments deep down inside and outwardly carry on quite well.

Our Father knows best. He knows that unforgiveness (like any other sin) harms us and other people. Our loving God doesn't want us to be hurt. He doesn't want us turned over to the torturers. (Matt. 18:34) He wants us healed and healthy in every way!

Jesus, is our great example of forgiving. Luke 23:34 records Him from the excruciating pain and rejection of the cross, crying out, "Father, forgive them; for they do not know what they are doing". The apostle Paul, in Eph. 4:32, warns we should be "forgiving each other, just as God in Christ also has forgiven you".

How many people, gnarled and hurting from arthritis are clinging to some old (or new) resentment, refusing to forgive one person for one slight? They may not know, or have forgotten that Jesus commanded us to forgive a person "seventy times seven", in Matt. 18:22. We see them in nursing homes, either neglected or perceiving they are. It can hurt to look at them, but they're the ones in pain, not the ones they haven't forgiven!

We can be offended in our daily activities. It could come from a parent, a sibling, son or daughter - anyone. Maybe it happened long ago and the hurter is long gone. No matter, we must forgive.

Not necessarily do we need to go to the person (if possible) face to face. That could dredge up old damage. And perhaps the other party isn't even aware of the situation.

Once, the Holy Spirit showed me I should forgive a boyhood buddy who seemed, while playing a game, intent on strangling another boy. I had forgotten all about it, but my Dad hadn't. So, decades later, I let it go.

Not only can healing and any type of deliverance be blocked by unforgiveness, but so can Heaven. Really? Look closely at the Lord's Prayer as well as Mark 11:26. You'll notice we don't get forgiven if we don't forgive. And if we don't get forgiven for our sins, guess what? Who are we, forgiven again and again by God, to refuse to forgive one or more trespasses against us? After all, we're children of God. Also, judging others and thereby playing God is none of our business!

I hadn't planned to devote a chapter to this subject, but the Lord constrained me to do it. Our loving God doesn't want us out of His will and His covenant!

Examples of easy does it

"When He (God) had disarmed the rulers and authorities, He made a public display of them having triumphed over them through Him (Jesus) (Colossians 2:15)

For years, Tess had pain from a pinched nerve in her lower back. She prayed, was believing God, but she still had pain. When she bent over, she knew that nerve was still pinching her.

But when we commanded a spirit of sciatica (pinched nerve) to leave, guess what? Tess bent and twisted and joyfully noticed there was no longer any pain.

Years of unnecessary suffering ended in seconds. The problem was easily identified, the solution was easily applied - a command to that spirit to leave in the name of Jesus. Any born-again Christian can do the same, for himself or someone else.

Yes, there can be garbage that has to be cleaned up first or that garbage (emotional spirits) can be the cause of the "infection", as we've noted earlier. Yet, so often, physical (and emotional) freedom can come from a single command in the name of the Lord.

Again and again, we will go into nursing homes and cast out deaf spirits (0ften inherited) and they will leave. Simple and quick. Unfortunately, too often, the party involved doesn't stand against the spirit's return by refusing it in the name of Jesus.

A lady from the East called us. She had a good report. After reading "God's Health Care Plan", she decided to come against an earache which was bothering her. She commanded it to leave in Jesus' name and she was freed from the earache. She had done what any believer can do. When Jesus said He came to give us a more abundant life, (John 10:10), He wasn't talking about Heaven.

Lorrie had pressure on her eyes. She was on the borderline of glaucoma. Several years before, a doctor, after checking her, suggested she "stay in touch". Lorrie didn't and the situation gradually deteriorated. From time she would also see halos of light in front of her. This demonic attack manifested strongly during one of our home meetings. The spirits were stirred up. But they would soon be gone.

We commanded, in this order, spirits of glaucoma, infirmity, blindness and pressure to leave in Jesus' name. Then we commanded the eye channels to open, the fluid to flow normally, and the scar tissue to be healed. After this was done, Lorrie reported the bothersome halos had left. Once we knew the problem, barely ten minutes were required. Incidentally, the pressure also left later.

One Saturday, when I was leaving a nursing home, I came to a couple of very nice ladies who had attended our bible studies there. One was a resident, the other a visitor. The latter lady revealed she had pain in her shoulder.

I commanded arthritis to leave, but she felt nothing except the continuing pain. Then I spoke to bursitis and tendonitis. It was short and sweet. Also, it served as a reminder that all muscular and bone aches aren't arthritis. Bursitis and tendonitis are also common - and as easy to cast out!

Millie had two sore heals. When she stood or walked, it hurt. At our Good News Church home bible fellowship, we commanded a variety of spirits to leave her, including a spirit of discomfort (describing what she was feeling). There was some relief.

However, a couple of weeks later, Millie reported she could stand and walk without pain. The Holy Spirit, honoring the name of Jesus, had completed the good work He'd begun in her. (Phil. 1:6)

Sometimes, a healing is not wholly manifested until later. Of course, the Lord can be expected to honor faith in His word and the name of Jesus every time. Since Jesus took Millie's pains long ago, she didn't have to go on bearing them herself!

At a woman's Christian retreat, Zelda, a non-Christian, was hurting. For years, she put up with vicious, out-of-the ordinary migraine headaches. She could vomit and be so oppressed she would retreat to into a dark room.

Also at the retreat was a Christian lady who offered to pray for Zelda. The two women left the meeting room and walked into the hall, stopping under the stairs. The second lady, who happened to be a new Christian, spoke an appropriate scripture, lay hands on the pain-filled lady, and commanded a spirit of pain to leave in the name of Jesus Christ.

Zelda reported the pain left her immediately. She was so impressed she went on to receive Jesus Christ as her Lord and Savior. Then she received the Baptism of the Holy Spirit. God ended years of agony in seconds - through the prayer of a new Christian. And that miracle led to two more miracles - the new birth and the Baptism of the Holy Spirit!

Jenni Spenner, a sophomore at Oral Roberts University, was news editor of the campus paper. One day, as she left the office with two associates, she missed a step. She heard her ankle snap and felt extreme pain.

Jennie saw the nurse. And the next morning, she was going to see the free doctor who would be on campus. Meanwhile, the pain was "horrible".

That night, Jenni long-distanced mom and dad, Art and Marilyn Spenner, at home in the Chicago area. They prayed and took authority over the ankle problem in the name of Jesus.

The next day, Jenni saw the doctor about her ankle. He told her there was "nothing wrong with it".The pain was gone and she was healed. A big deal for appreciative Jenni. No big deal for a too-seldom - appreciated God.

Child-like faith is most easily found in children. Even in today's sophisticated world system, they're more likely to be untouched by doubt. Take Jeremy. At the age of ten, he still believes his mother - and God. So when his family was staying in semi-primitive quarters during a summer vacation and Jeremy was sleeping in the loft , the boy was set free from a particular fear. What was it? Jeremy felt "spooked" up in that loft at night. Discovering Jeremy's apprehension, mom told him to tell that scared feeling to go away, that Jesus was protecting him.

Jeremy did it, the feeling left and he fell asleep more easily. He's been taught to use that powerful name of Jesus. And he uses it!

Even successful people need help. A very capable,likeable and popular talk-show hostess was glad to get prayer. And in a few minutes, Jesus Christ delivered her from tension and stress, anxiety, occult curses and a controlling spirit. She then felt a new peace - the kind the world can't give but everyone in the world can use.

You might be surprised at whom God would bless through you - and how easy it can be, especially if He sets it up.

One day, I called one of our credit card providers for information. After receiving it, I felt I should witness to the young lady on the phone. When I did, I discovered she was a Christian and had diabetes. She wanted prayer. So, anxiety and fear were cast out. Others that left were imbalance spirits, including sugar imbalance. (The imbalance demons seemed logical targets, given the diabetes.) A spirit of diabetes was also spoken to.

The young lady felt better, "more relaxed". She could have lost the diabetes. I don't know. But I do know she was happier at the end of the short, maybe four minute session.

You can do the same. In fact, helping people through simple deliverance should be the norm for every true Christian. The opportunities are everywhere. And the Holy Spirit is inside every born-again Christian!

In Illinois, there are many mental health type nursing homes. Manic depression and schizophrenia are common among the residents, most of are male.

Bud is a youngish man who often comes at our church bible study at his nursing home. His major problem seems to be manic depression. He's had for close to thirty years. One Saturday, we were able to help him. Realizing he had a restless spirit, Bud accepted prayer. We suggested this time he take authority himself. When he commanded a spirit of restlessness to leave in Jesus' name, he felt relaxed. Then he commanded a spirit of depression to leave. More good news. To his pleasant surprise, he felt even more relaxed. The spirits are subject to Bud. (Luke 10:20)

Martin Halwix enjoyed playing basketball. The 17-year-old senior was a starter on his high-school team. The 1996-97 season was about to begin, but Martin wasn't about to play.

A vertebra problem that began years earlier had burst forth and was bringing constant pain. What a chiropractor had uncovered, including a pinched nerve in the back, would sorely affect his senior year in high school.

But God is always on time. The chiropractor had noted that Martin's right leg was about an inch shorter than the left leg. The back problem resulted.

As Martin sat flush against the back of a chair, Faye, held his legs out, commanded a spirit of infirmity to leave his back, and she commanded parts of the back to relax and align. Then she told the right leg to grow out - all, of course, in the name of Jesus.

The change was visible. The length of both legs seemed now to be the same. Martin stood, touched his toes and sway-bent his back more than once. No question that all of the pain was gone. He was free to play basketball. Total timing for God's healing - less than five minutes. That's less than it takes for five time outs!

Postscript. One of Martin's parents called several weeks later. Two trips to the chiropractor had confirmed that Martin was totally healed. No more trips were planned.

One of our grand-daughters, aged 4 1/2, came into our house in sad shape. She had fallen on her tailbone and it hurt. But with grandma holding her close, grandpa commanded a spirit of infirmity to leave that area and also told the muscles, ligaments, nerves , vertebrae and discs in the back to come into proper alignment.

The young lady, who had been twisting her body, uncomfortably, now twisted it more comfortably.

Sometimes, people feel so much better, they may not be concerned when some of the pain remains. That afternoon, we discovered this was the case with our grand-daugter. So, we again spoke to the same spirits and parts. This time, she could bend over and she reported the pain was gone. Jesus had completed the work.

Phil was scheduled for surgery. He had an 80% hearing loss in one ear and a loss of 75% in the other.The day before he was scheduled to be checked by the doctor, Phil was hoping to get prayer in a specific Christian meeting, but he wasn't able to make it.

Knowing his Lord wasn't limited to church buildings and special meetings, Phil took things into his own hands.Literally. He laid his hands on his ears and took authority in the name of Jesus Christ.

The next day, at his doctor's office, a checkup indicated his hearing loss had been reduced to 30% in each ear. The doctor cancelled surgery.

Two weeks later, testing showed only a 5% hearing loss remained. Shortly after that, Phil's ears popped. Now there was no more hearing loss at all. The percentage that God prefers is 100%!

From time to time, I'll realize there's a Christian song running through my mind, over and over. It's not from God, but from a spirit of religion. Possibly this occurs because I was once delivered from such a spirit. The song might be "Amazing Love", "Gentle Jesus", etc. - fine songs. But not when there's something driving about them. The Holy Spirit is gentle.

What do I do? If I'm not sure of the source, I'll test the spirit. First John 4:2 tells us , "every spirit that confesses Jesus Christ has come in the flesh is from God". So I can ask the spirit, in the name of Jesus, if it believes Jesus came in the flesh. If the mental song leaves, I know it's from a demonic source.

However, since this is not the same as rebuking, the song seems to return quickly. The way to drive it out, period, is to command it leave, in the name of Jesus.

If you ever get harassed by this kind of stuff, don't stand for iat. For your peace of mind, drive it out in Jesus' name!

We shouldnt put up with a fever, or anything else in our kids. Jesus took their sicknesses and pains as well as ours..

Speaking on the phone with a friend, we learned the young daughter was ill and had a fever. So, as mom laid hands on her, we commanded the spirit of fever to leave and did the same for influenza and any other spirit of infirmity. The girl then reported feeling "hot". The fever was going and so was the problem it heralded. The Lord loves children. He still wants them brought to Him, so He can lay hands on them and bless them.

Our young-adult niece likes to baby-sit for her nieces. This can include a certain amount of lifting and piggy-back hauling. That can bring back pain. And that can also increase any pain you've had for a nunber of years.

When we prayed for her,we spoke to several spirits with no success. Then, we decided to do "the pelvis thing". She stood, feet apart and Faye, our specialist in such things, took over. As I was commanding any spirit of infirmity to leave her back, Faye put her hands on our niece's hips and commanded the pelvis to relax and get into proper alignment. The Holy Spirit then moved the young lady gently around for about five minutes. Then, she checked her back. There was no more pain.

In brief minutes, Jesus Christ had freed our niece from pain. That's probably far less time than even the drive to your friendly chiropractor.

One of Myra's eyes was a mess. It was hurting and dilated. She had gone to a physician who guessed a virus was causing the pain and inconvenience. With eye drops, the eye was dilated. But the pain remained. It was a nuisance.

However, when a fellow Christian commanded spirits of eye infirmity and pain out in the name of Jesus, Myra felt the power of God. She also knew the pain was gone. Viruses are demonic, so they (or what's behind them) must bend the knee to the name which is above all names. They have no choice.

God doesn't fool around. He doesn't want us to, either. He wants to heal people and to that end makes things as easy as possible for us to do our small part.

Evidences of spirits leaving

"'Now when the unclean spirit has gone out of a man..." (Matthew 12:43)

How do we know when an evil spirit leaves someone? Obviously, when a disease goes away, the causative spirit or spirits have departed. A simple example is a headache. No more headache, no more spirit. With deafness, the command is given, the spirit leaves, the ears are open. Sometimes,. the cold you've prayed against may not be gone until the next morning. Then, the involved spirit surely should also be gone, further healing may have also taken place.

But, when emotional spirits go, how are we aware of it? Well, if someone who had stress becomes relaxed, that's a pretty sure indication. Or, when anger subsides, or a depressed person perks up, that's a pretty certain indication. Very often, the deliveree may not feel 100% better when one spirit departs. So, we should know what else to look for, to ask about, in order to discern what other spirit should be addressed - do it - and watch for results.

Spirits can leave in a number of ways. The Greek word" pneuma" literally means "breath" and can figuratively mean "demon". Many spirits are breathed out. Sometimes, it's with sigh, a yawn , a sharp expelling of air, a cough, even a deep breath or belching.

Yet, there are many other evidences of demon departure: a lightness, a feeling of something lifting or leaving, a warmth, coolness, tingling, a sudden smile, laughter, crying or sobbing - and yes, there can be vomiting. We have never encountered the latter ourselves. Why? Perhaps because we usually bind Satan when we begin deliverance. Here are a few varied examples.

Seth told us, as we prayed and he was being delivered

from a group of spirits (one at a time), that most often the release seemed to be "things" leaving straight up out of his head. Feeling better and sharper was the outcome.

A feeling of release seems quite common. Personally, I experienced a tremendous release in my gut when the Holy Spirit drove out a long-held pious religious spirit. To make sure I got the message, the Lord showed me, in an open vision, a small, unpleasant-appearing pious spirit, whose legs went into slipper-like feet. It tiptoed across my vision and off the screen. A vision, with me, has not been the norm. I've been released from quite a few other spirits and never have seen any of them.

A man with digestive problems felt something lift when we cast out a spirit of chemical imbalance. With the loss of a spirit of biochmemical imbalance, he said something seemed to leave his arms. After the expulsion of about a dozen spirits, he, as so many others, experienced a strong peace.

A lady, whose chest problem was very emotionally-induced, cried when several strong spirits left. Other manifestations included coughing. Most of the pain was gone at the end of the session and surgery wasn't necessary.

Laughter seems to sometimes come on when a spirit of low body self image comes out. One lady who had that spirit reported that after it left, she felt as if she wanted to laugh. First, she felt a cracking in her neck.

A man in a nursing home commented he felt like something left him when a spirit of depression was commanded to go.

I seem to have a constant battle with spirits of anxiety. A yawn, deep breath, or physical slumping can occur when I take authority over those spirits. Anxiety, I believe, was inherited from my mother, who toughed it out during the depression. And, I most likely picked it up as a child. So, addressing childhood and inherited spirits of anxiety is proving helpful. (See Chapter 16 on the categories of spirits.)

James was delivered from several spirits including anger. Each time he reported feeling warmth. Why? Perhaps God was showing His love to His son who was trying very hard to be more Christ-like. The outward result? His temper was less evident at home.

Rhonda was afraid of her husband. She felt release when spirits of fear of rejection and hopelessness left her.

A man ,delivered from years of drug addiction, felt bathed in the power of God when the spirits were driven out. Near the end of the session, he cried at times and also felt the warmth of the Holy Spirit.

Faye, in battling anxiety and kindred spirits, can experience an almost gurgling belch.

What's most important is not how spirits go but that they do go. Yet, it certainly helps the person or persons delivering themselves or others to realize God works in many ways - and be able to recognize a manifestation. Usually, evidence of demon departures are no big deal with retching and thrashing on the floor, etc. Yes, that can happen, and when and if it does, you'll know!

Spirits, who try to live and exhibit their personalities through their hosts, may manifest those personalities before they have been cast out. I was present when a spirit of theatrics came on someone who kept rushing at people in the room. It wasn't until a member of the deliverance team received a word of knowledge from the Holy Spirit that the spirit of theatrics was identified and cast out. Theatrics also proved to be the blocker to the expulsion of other spirits.

A man, after being delivered from four or five long-time enemies, still wasn't totally free. At last, a spirit manifested and the man's jaws moved as if he were viciously going after a piece of meat in a very primitive fashion. The spirit was power. When it was then addressed, it was powerless and had to leave! That wonderful name of Jesus! That session, I might add, helped turn that man's life around.

Jesus said in Luke 11:20, "But if I cast out spirits by the finger (Spirit) of God, then the kingdom of God has come upon you". The written word of God gives us the following definition of the Kingdom of God (Romans 14:17), "for the kingdom of God is righteousness, peace and joy in the Holy Spirit".

No wonder so many set free by Jesus through the Holy Spirit feel a new peace after old things have passed away!

Back and respiratory problems take off

"The power of the Lord was present to heal them." (Luke 5:17 KJV)

The most common physical problems are in backs and upper respiratory systems. A 1996 chiropractic publication states that 8 out of every 10 Americans suffer from recurrent back pain. The cost of workers' compensation is close to $20 billion per year.

Upper and lower back pain, scoliosis, disc, joint and vertebrae problems are surprisingly common. However, first place is held by head colds, sinusitis, sore throats, bronchitis, etc. Who hasn't heard of or suffered from "the common cold"? Yet, like all other diseases, they're caused by demons who must give place in the name of Jesus!

Back problems

Looking back on long-term lower back problems, I vividly recall being set free at an area bible study. My shorter left leg grew out and out went the back pain and off could come the heel lifts from my left shoes.

In September, 1996, a radio show host reported lower back pain. That's usually a cinch for the Lord.

Sitting in a chair and extending his legs out, the host noticed one leg was shorter than the other. The healing procedure? Command any spirit of infirmity to leave the back; command every muscle, ligament, nerve, disc, tendon and vertebra to move into proper alignment. Then, command the short leg to grow out. All, of course, in the name of Jesus.

As we did this, the back pain left this dedicated voice of Christian radio. Sounds like Jesus operating in His authority in one of the gospels, doesn't it? Truth is, the Lord is still doing it. Remember, Jesus Christ is "the same, yesterday and today, yes and forever". He'll do the same thing for you as He did for that radio show host. Because He is also still "no respecter of persons". (Rom. 2:11)

Jeff had lower back pain. His chiropractor had indicated sciatica was involved. His right leg was about 1/4" shorter than the left. First, we commanded spirits of sciatica and scoliosis to leave.Then we spoke to infirmity, told areas of the back to relax and align and the right leg to grow out. The leg grew out. Jeff felt better - and even better when a spirit left his back. The total procedure took only a few minutes and ended the necessity of constant visits to the doctor. God is very able!

What about a lower back problem? You, or the party involved, stand straight and extend both arms out until the hands are almost clapped together. Notice which arm is shorter and after commanding a spirit of infirmity to leave the back, command every muscle, ligament, nerve, vertebra, disc and tendon to relax and align align properly. Finally, command the short arm to grow out - all in the name of Jesus.

Bob had a leadership position with his organization. He was a busy man. And he was hampered by a deteriorating hip that was arthritic. A Christian, he was open for prayer during the phone conversation.

When a spirit of arthritis was commanded to leave, nothing seemed to transpire. But, all pain left when inflammation, pain and swelling were cast out.

Often, back (and other problems), are solved by what the Hunters call "the pelvis thing". The hips (pelvis) are cleared of any spirit of infirmity, the pelvis is commanded to rotate into proper alignment, also in the name of Jesus. As this was done with Bob, the Holy Spirit began moving his body around to perform what was necessary to complete the work He had begun. Now, we did end the call. Hip rotating may take quite a while - and we were on long distance! Though, there is no distance in the spirit world where the Lord reigns supreme.

Here's a case of lower back pain - plus. On a night in 1996, Faye, checked the length of Ginny's legs. One leg was at least an inch shorter than the other. We cast out a spirit of sciatica and any spirit of infirmity from her back, also speaking to parts of her back to relax and come into alignment, speaking to parts of the back also. The short leg grew out and Ginny felt improvement. But there was still stiffness, so we cast out a spirit of stiffness. The back felt much better.

Someone also noted one of Ginny's hips bones was higher than the other. Then we did "the pelvis thing". As Faye laid hands on Ginny's pelvis, the Holy Spirit began moving her body. After a matter of minutes, the movement stopped and Ginny was more improved. Both hip bones were now at the same height.

That wasn't the end of it. The Lord likes us totally free. Ginny had a sore shoulder. As I recall, we drove off spirits of arthritis, bursitis and tendonitis. Then the soreness was gone. Isn't it reassuring to know that Jesus, in Himself, has restored the authority that God gave to man in the days of Adam? (Gen. 1:26)

The spine affects much of the body, even organs. Ask a chiropractor, he can tell you how important it is. That's why "the pelvis thing" and lengthening arms and legs can even affect more than legs, arms and hips.

In January, 1996, Liz had broken her back. Her first vertebra was crushed. In November, she was walking, but she didn't go long distances or stand for any period of time. It was too painful.

Liz called for prayer. And our omnipresent God was present across the miles. On the phone, a fellow lay person took authority in the name of Jesus. First, a spirit of accident injury trauma was cast out of her back. Liz felt a tickling in her body. She hurt less. Then the vertebrae and other back parts were commanded into proper alignment; healing was commanded. Now, the pressure was gone. Inflammation was cast out and Liz felt even better. There was no reaction to a spirit of soreness, but when swelling was driven out, she felt "like a lifting". The pain was all gone. In about ten minutes, Jesus Christ had healed another one of His people!

Respiratory problems

In upper respiratory situations, we often speak to a chain of spirits. Depending on the problem, these can include laryngitis, pharyngitis, sinusitis, catarrh, post-nasal drip, bronchial asthma and bronchitis - inherited, allergic "or otherwise". This covers the waterfront. (Pun intended.)

Laura was allergic to dust and pollen and prone to bronchial asthma. After residual spirits left her, we spoke to the "sinus chain", beginning with sinusitis., Her nasal passages began clearing. She could breathe better.

It sounds simple, doesn't it? Well, driving out spirits often is. The reason is not us. God's mighty power is constantly available at the mighty name of Jesus!

Mike had chronic sinus problems. When we talked with him, he sounded in the middle of one. But God is an expert in bringing light that dissipates darkness and power that clears up sinuses. We took authority over spirits of sinusitis, allergic rhinitis, catarrh, bronchitis and bronchial asthma - inherited, allergic or otherwise. And we commanded the passages to open.

Mike felt relief immediately. His sinuses opened. Yet, there remained that long-term allergy problem. But, when inherited allergy spirits were evicted, Mike felt a tingling in the center of his body. (Tingling is one manifestation of the Holy Spirit.) God moved on that allergy.

For ten days, Kerry had upper respiratory disease. A dry cough hacked away at her. She was breathing with difficulty.

But, her church turned out to be her promised land. She wanted prayer and wanted to feel better. Both expectations came about.

One of the staff members began taking authority. Kerry was in stress, so that spirit was dispatched. Then several others were driven out including an inherited spirit of fear.The last step was a command, in the name of Jesus, for the inherited spirit of bronchial asthma to leave her. Kerry reported the dryness and breathing difficulty were no more. The full process covered from five to ten minutes.

Headaches are often caused by sinus problems. These, we find, are usually inherited. Mom, dad, aunt, uncle, etc. could have had them. And those spirits cling to the family vine.

When Alise called, she was having another headache, not a migraine, but the discomfort that comes from a sinus infection. At the time her sinuses felt stuffy.

In the name of Jesus, we commanded inherited spirits of sinusitis, allergic rhinitis, catarrh and post nasal drip to leave Alise. She reported her left sinus was clearing and her head felt better. God wants our heads clear, in more ways than one!

Steve Chapman is an Evansville, Indiana broadcaster who loves God a lot. And the feeling is mutual. One day in 1995, while speaking by phone with Steve, I was able to pray against his (really the devil's) long-term bronchitis and laryngitis - not exactly assets for an announcer.

Over a year later, Steve reported that after that prayer of authority, he has had no more signs of bronchitis or laryngitis. His work for God, in and out of the station, could go on unhindered!

As a child, and in military service, I had sinus problems. Nose drops became a common medication for me. As a Christian, I've been successfully able to fend off sinusitis, rhinitis, etc. But, I've discovered it's important to stay on top of them. It shouldn't have to be necessary to pour in nose drops, take anti-histamines and so on. These things don't solve anything. They're only temporary palliatives - and they can cause an unhealthy dependency.

The answer is the Lord Who heals you. With Him, these stories - and your story - can have a happy ending.

Moral to these accounts: don't back off from fighting back against back problems or respiratory raids - and they'll get off of you or whoever you"re praying for!

Conquests of cancer heart disease and death

"This day the Lord will deliver you up into my hands, and I will strike you down" *(I Samuel 1:46)*

Maybe you've heard it said it's one thing to have faith for God to heal a head cold and another to trust Him to drive out a more dread disease. Possibly. But remember, that WHO you have faith in is more important than what you have faith for.

The apostle Paul, who had what you might call anti-faith in Jesus before he was apprehended on the Damascus Road, later said, "I know Whom I have believed". (I Tim. 1:12) As a Christian, you should know the Lord and that He wants you to know the power of His resurrection.

Matthew 4:23 informs us Jesus was healing every kind of sickness among the people. (KJV) There were no exceptions. And Hebrews 13:8 reminds us He's the same today as He was yesterday.

It also helps to remember you're not doing the healing, He is!

Cancer

Ulyses Anderson was ninety years old. He was a firm believer with a healthy outlook on life. In all his years, his only medication was aspirin.

Then the destroyer did his best. He hit Ulyses with prostate cancer, the most common cancer in males and most commonly a killer. After x-rays and biopsy indicated malignancy, surgery was called for. But, when Ulyses was opened up, the severely swollen condition of his prostate was evident. This, plus his advanced age, contra-indicated surgery. The outlook

wasn't very hopeful. Especially considering U
from cancer.

Most afflictees in such a situation woul
Not Ulyses, his son or daughter. Knowing
the name of Jesus, his offspring did what they kne.
They laid hands son their dad and commanded the cancer and other appropriate spirits to get out in the name of Jesus Christ.

Another x-ray and biopsy were taken. Two days after the doctors had opened and closed Ulyses' body, one of the physicians told son and daughter, "I can't understand it". Those latest tests showed no signs of cancer or need to go further. Even the bleeding had stopped. Ulyses was healed. At ninety, he went home and went on with life. And, there was great joy in his family!

Jesus would like to satisfy you with long life, too, as Psalm 91 promises, and show you His salvation.

Pastor John McCall's church is appropriately called Baltimore Christian Faith Center. And John McCall puts his faith on the line, again and again.

Some years ago, a lady in the church was diagnosed with cancer. Tests showed she had 29 cancerous lymph nodes on one breast. Not exactly a joyous revelation.

When she came to church, Pastor McCall took authority over that totally demonic mess in the name of Jesus Christ. The moment of truth came on the operating table. The patient's body was opened; it was closed. How come? There was nothing there, not even a node.

All was well for ten years. Then the devil struck again and delivered three breast tumors, each larger than a marble. Our lady went through x-rays, mammogram and MRI. The signs were unmistakable. The necessary procedure was surgery.

But, that wasn't necessary. This time by telephone, Pastor McCall took authority in the name of Jesus over a spirit of infirmity and cursed the cancer from the roots.

Later, a mammogram and x-rays showed not a single lump was left. And, very soon, the lady left the hospital.

Not all healing stories have such a happy ending. Consider Marty. She went to a meeting of two well-known healing evangelists. An unbeliever, she was completely healed of cancer. Then she became a believer in Jesus Christ. How could she doubt He'd been raised from the dead? And she was turned on for God.

Years later, the devil returned with another package of cancer. Unfortunately, Marty no longer had that simple faith and trust in the Lord. She had become a proudly active Christian. That may have been part of the problem. Perhaps the Lord now expected more from her than in her pre-Christian days and early Christian babyhood.

The sad ending is that Marty died of cancer. The devil would probe our weak spots, and if our defences aren't up, we could go down!

Sarcoidosis is vicious. This demon calcifies lung tissue and can cause instant blindness and/or heart stoppage. So, who needs it? Certainly not the 34-year-old lady who was terminally afflicted with it.

Let's call her Robin. She came to a Steve Sampson meeting in the Canadian province of New Brunswick. She came expecting to be healed - even though, a Christian, she had never visited such a church before.

The last night of meetings arrived. By the time the service was nearly over, God had still not healed a dismayed Robin. Then, at the last minute, the Lord spoke through Steve Sampson. He called out the problem. Then Steve and others prayed and Steve cast out the cancer spirit.

Healing was instantaneous. Robin felt better. The next day, she and friends left for a short vacation on Prince Edward Island. Instead of lying across the back seat, Robin drove all the way. When she arrived, she phoned Steve and told him what had happened. A subsequent trip to the doctor and more testing proved the terminal cancer had been terminated. Nearly all of the scar tissue had disappeared. That was in 1994. Two years later, Robin continued to flourish. Cancer free!

In June of 1996, Steve Sampson was ministering in Knoxville, Tennessee. A lady at the meeting had sarcoidosis. She was also hard of hearing.

When Steve related the above-noted healing in New Brunswick, the lady, not hearing correctly, thought he had given a word of knowledge for her. And she received it as such. Result - God healed her. Not only did the sarcoidosis leave, but her hearing returned!

The Lord is looking for faith, and when He finds it, He'll move. And, He even overlooks mistakes!

Heart Disese

Poverbs 4:23 warns us to watch over our hearts with all diligence, because out of them come the issues of life. Normally, that scripture refers to guarding our spirits. Nevertheless, it makes sense in the physical, too. Our hearts are centrol to our continuing existence. They stop and we stop.

Dr. Tom, a dentist in his sixties, discovered the left ventricle of his heart was enlarged. He was diagnosed with Ekocardiosis. A a bible warrior, he cursed the problem, received authoritative prayer, spoke to his heart daily and confessed healing and restoration, thanking God. He was very diligent.

After a few months, Dr.Tom underwent an Eko stress test that revealed the condition of his heart valves. He passed the test and discovered the heart problem had passed away. In the words of his cardiologist, "you don't have it".

Take heart, you don't have to have it, either.

Death

Jesus, in Matthew 10:8, commanded His apostles to raise the dead. In Matthew 5:41, the Lord raised a 12-year-old girl from death. And in the 14th Chapter of John, He states that we who believe in Him would do the works He did.

A Missouri pastor did just that. A young girl, not yet in

her teens, had been run over and killed by an ongoing vehicle. It happened outside of and after church on Sunday. The ambulance had been called and was on the way.

Quite a few minutes after the deadly accident, the pastor came out to the street. (His was a storefront church.) He took the limp child into his arms. There was no pulse.

Then the compassionate pastor prayed and felt God was telling him to call forth the spirit of life. As I recall his testimony, he bound the devil or spirit of death - then he did command the spirit of life to return to the girl.

Almost immediately, she opened her eyes. Her pulse, her life, returned. And the pastor could restore her to her parents, just as Jesus did in Matthew 5:41.

The spirit of life in Jesus Christ has set us free from the law of sin and death (Romans 8:2)!

The bookstore lady who wins

> **"God chose the weak things of the world to shame the strong ."**
> **(I Corinthians 1:27 NIV)**

We know a lady who never went to bible school, and never sat under a great Christian teacher, but she's strong in the Lord and the power of His might. In fact, where once she was weak, she's now filled with holy boldness. The devil is no match for her because she knows who she is and what she has in Christ. Yet, it wasn't always that way.

Today's she's a healthy middle-aged great-grandmother. But when she was in her thirties, her physician predicted she would dead by age 34. A dismaying prognosis.

She walked around with super ventricular tacchardia.Her heartbeat was racing. Her heart was wearing out. In case that weren't enough, the devil had hit her with a rare form of hemophilia, a blood disease that prevents the buildup of red blood cells. Her medication included a very heavy 40 mg dosage of enderol three times a day. On top of the above, she had a severely arthritic back. Satan had come to rob, kill and destroy her. Perhaps he could see what would happen if he didn't do it.

Spiritually, she wasn't very healthy, either. She had become a backslider, moved away from Jesus Christ.

One day, as she was reading her Bible in the New Mexico countryside, where her husband worked on a petroleum pipeline, Jesus intervened in her life. An audible voice spoke clearly to her as she was reading Revelation 3:15. "so because you are lukewarm, I will spit you out of my mouth". The voice said. "that's you, and if you don't repent, I'm going to vomit you out of my mouth!" Her version of the Bible didn't state "vomit", but when she looked it up in the Greek, sure enough, it was "vomit".

That word from the Lord, our lady recalls, changed the course of her life. She decided to live for Jesus. Not only did she increase her praying and Bible reading and make personal changes, she reached for more of God.

At a later date, she went to the altar of a church to receive the Baptism of the Holy Spirit (Acts 1:5, 1:8, Mark 16:7). When the pastor lay his hands on her, she saw a white light coming down and into her body. The arthritis and years of pain were gone. Her heart stopped racing. Tests also proved the blood disease had disappeared. As a bonus, the Lord took away her desire for cigarets. (She'd been a chain smoker since her teens.)

Today, many years later, she's a picture of health and runs a bookstore in Branson, Missouri. And - this proprietess casts out demons and sees God heal local residents and those in town for vacations. Let's look at some cases.

Post-Partem Depression

Quite noticeably, Corinne was in the bookstore. She was sobbing and distraught. Why? Post-partem depression. She'd been in this super-blues state for the eight month period since she'd delivered her baby. She was on the brink of suicide.

Doctors didn't have the answer, but God did. And the owner, who long since has ceased to be lukewarm, prayed right then and there. During her prayer, she realized there was a spirit of post-partem depression. And she went for it. In the name of Jesus Christ, she angrily commanded that gloom-and-doom spirit to leave her customer. She had no doubt it would go - and it did. The result was eye-boggling. Corinne's countenance changed. She smiled. Employees said she wasn't the same person. Jesus Christ had broken eight months of bondage.

Corinne walked out of that bookstore with much more than she'd bargained for. But God promises in the Third Chapter of Ephesians, Verse 20, that He is "able to do exceedingly beyond all we ask or think".

Degenerative Muscle Disease

When Phil visited the bookstore,he was on total disability Afflicted with degenerative muscle disease, he couldn't work. Phil didn't relish his situation, so he agreed to prayer Our bookstore lady went after the caue of it all. She commanded appropriate spirits to leave her customer in the name of Jesus Christ. Phil's head bent back; he seemed to be in a back bend. "I can't breathe", he cried. But Becky continued taking authority in the name of the Lord. And the demonic grip came loose. New strength came into Phil. He walked out a new person.

The following Thursday, Phil went into the hospital for testing. he was told there was nothing wrong with him. He was taken off disability. At last, Phil was free to work. Demons had disabled him, but God enabled him to lead the more abundant life Jesus came to bring him. (John 10:10)

Emphysema and Tumors

When it comes to healing, or anything else, God is no respecter of persons. (Acts 10:34) He'll heal one as well as the other.Consider what happened in a local hospital room.

Our bookstore lady was visiting the 13-year-old son of a friend. The boy, filling with tumors throughout his body, had gained 200 pounds and at the time weighed 300 pounds. The lady asked if he would like prayer.

Overhearing, the man in the other bed spoke up. "You cann pray for me, too", he volunteered. He was hospitalized for emphysema. So our lady laid hands on him and commanded a spirit of emphysema to leave him in the name

of Jesus. Then, she returned to the teenager. For him, she cursed the tumors, commanded them to be dried up and said "be healed", in the name of Jesus. Then she left.

The next day, the boy with tumors and the man with emphysema were tested. The boy had no more tumors. The man had no more emphysema. Both were dismissed from the hospital. All because our God is an awesome God and, as He promised, "all things are possible to him who believes". (Mark 9:23)

Is the lady in Branson special? No. She's just one more born-again Christian who knows what to do and does it. So, God is with her, time after time. What she does, you, fellow Christian, can do also!

Christian cooperation pays off

"For the body is not one member, but many"
(I Corinthians 12:14)

Jesus is the vine, we are the branches. He is the head, we are the body. Notice that "we" in there. Even the Lone Ranger had Tonto, so he wasn't really a lone ranger.

The chuch (ecclesia) is composed of God's called out people. One calling we all have is to call on the name of Jesus and go out and set the captives free. And in these last days, God wants all hands on deck, so He's eager to shape up His troops.

Very often, we're called to work together to dislodge the enemy - and always called to learn from each other and share what we know.

Diane Wirth is a quick learner filled with holy boldness and Christ-like compassion. Diane, her daughter and her husband have all been healed through commanding prayer in the name of Jesus. So, Diane went and did likewise. When she called for supporting prayer for a lady in a hospital, we discovered that on an earlier occasion she took her Jesus-given authority on behalf of someone else, and experienced results.

What happened? In speaking to someone on the phone, Diane discovered the lady had a tumor on her chest. And Diane knew exactly what to do. First, she had the other lady (a Christian) lay a hand on the area of the growth. Then Diane commanded the spirit to go, in the name of Jesus. And - the tumor was gone, she excitedly reported. It had left immediately.

Diane had learned from her own healings, used what she had learned and utilized the prayee in the process. Of course, Jesus healed, confirming His word with signs following.

What word? In Mark 16, He promises that believers, in His name, would lay hands on the sick who in turn would recover.

That's not all. While we were talking with Diane, she told us her young-adult daughter had fallen and cut her eye and eyelid. It was painful and the young lady was feeling miserable. Then we did what we knew - commanded any spirits of break or cut to leave and did the same with pain, inflammation, infection and blindness. Result - the pain left, the girl looked and felt better. Mother was happy. Daughter was happy. We were happy. And, I believe Jesus was happy because the girl was healed and through other members of His body.

Even that's not all. The next day, Diane, in happy tears, called to report that her daughter was totally healed. No more cuts in the eye area. She had opened her eyes after three days from the fall and was joyfully amazed. Our God is a good God!

Why didn't Diane pray for her daughter? Perhaps she was too upset. Maybe her daughter didn't have faith in her own mother. Sometimes it can take someone outside of the family to do it. That's where fellow believers can step in. It's the Holy Spirit Who does the work, not any of us.

Look at that wonderful word, "believers" - it's plural and refers to every member of the body of Christ. Not just evangelists, pastors or special people. It encompasses all of us - Christian soldiers enrolled in the same army!

God's word tells Christians to encourage one another. And it does make a difference. At the Chicago area's Rosemont Horizon, we'd spoken to a fellow layman from Good News Church. He mentioned growing out a limb for someone right there in the seats.

So, when the opportunity arose during a Christian meeting at the same huge indoor facility, we seized it. The man had experienced upper and lower back pain for years. But, in the name of Jesus, (Who took that pain on His own back), his years of uneccesary suffering would end.

One of his legs was shorter than the other. The prescription was (as he held his legs out from a sitting position) to command a spirit of infirmity to leave the back and tell each part of the back (vertebrae, discs, etc) to come into proper alignment - then to command the short leg to grow out. The result was predictable. The man's leg grew out and the lower back pain left.

Checking comparaative arm lengths indicated one limb was shorter than the other. The same commanding procedure (in Jesus' name) (this time to the back and short arm) brought the same kind of result - no more upper back pain. The total time for both operations was about ten minutes. Only God could do that!

But the happy ending couldn't have been written had not one member of Jesus' body been encouragement to another member.

There are times when one of God's people seems to have no one to turn to for help. How can that happen with so many Christians around? Well, if you live in a small community and go around constantly ministering to other people, you may have a problem finding someone knowledgeable enough to pray for you.

Marcia is a broadcaster who prays for people and teaches them on and off the air. She had been crying out to God to send someone to help. In preparing to call for telephone interviews, I spotted (in the Broadcasting Red Book) a Christian station in a very small city. Normally, I prefer larger cities. But I did pray and surprisingly got a release to call this station. I did and Marcia received the help she needed. The Lord has His own network.

God has His timing. Most Spirit-led Christians experience it often in their own lives. For example, here's how I became scheduled on a certain Christian station.

One Friday afternoon, I decided to recall a program host who had spoken weeks earlier about calling me to interview on "God's Health Care Plan". When I reached him, he commented that earlier in the day he had pulled up my material and placed it on the top of the pile on his desk. He planned to call me, but hadn't done it. Now, our timing meshed and we booked the interview. The Holy Spirit will move on members of the Body of Christ when He wills.

Sometimes people need help, but they don't attend a church that believes in divine healing and/or deliverance, or can handle it properly. This was the case with Verna. She had been depressed and had marital problems. She had received prayer more than once, gone to a counselor - not much help. Fortunately, Verna had a close friend who wanted to see her set free by Jesus Christ. She called Faye and I, and we in turn contacted Verna. Three members of the body helping the fourth.

Questioning and the leading of the Holy Spirit revealed deep problems. One was the hurt and guilt of an abortion years earlier, before she became a Christian. This time, on the phone, Verna lost a few spirits that made her life miserable. Among them were stress, worry, depression and guilt.

An abortion, no matter how long ago, means heartache, hurt, guilt and self-condemnation. No matter how inexpensive the surgical procedure, the ongoing cost can be unbearable. Also, we learned there was a spirit of perfectionism and cast it out.

By the end of her deliverance, Verna was different inside. No longer depressed and filled with other destructive spirits gnawing on her, she had been freed by Jesus Christ - and she knew it. What tremendous satisfaction to be a part of Jesus' body on earth and see the Lord move to change lives!

There's usually an air of expectancy at our home bible fellowship. We never know what God is going to do and through whom. We've learned He often uses many of His members to help one hurting member.,

Max attended one of these home services in 1996. When personal prayer time arrived, he told us he had important decisions to make and wanted guidance from the Lord.

Conversation revealed that Max was fearful. He had an inherited spirit of fear and also fear of sickness. (Although he was healthy, he had a long-time fear of becoming ill.) Anxiety was dispatched, followed panic and terror. As the commanding prayer continued, Max was experiencing increasing peace. He had felt rejected and held the fear of it happening again. So those spirits were driven out. And throughout the deliverance, the Holy Spirit was informing different people to help move things along properly.

Max told us he was never satisfied with his efforts. That meant a driving spirit had to go, and it did. Resentment and anger were next. Then someone received a word of knowledge - chemical imbalance. At the command, Max felt something lift and leave him. (He had been taking enzymes for digestive difficulties.) Biochemical imbalance and hormanal imbalance departed. Metabolic imbalance did the same - and Max knew it

When Max left that night, he had a new peace within him. Evil spirits can cause turmoil -and Max had it. But as Jesus worked through His members, He once again showed Himself as the Prince of Peace!

Several months later, Max, smiling and happy, wanted prayer for himself and his bride-to-be. He reported he was still free from that old driving spirit and was able to function more relaxedly. Yes, he did use the list we had given him of the spirits God had delivered him from.

Whom the Lord will use at these meetings is up to him, not us. One night, one of the ladies had a heavy anointing in her hands. They felt hot. And she was able to lay hands on people there with results. Another night, the Lord led someone to lay hands on everyone in the room - and three of them burst into holy laughter.

"Where the Spirit of the Lord is there is fredom." (2 Cor. 3:17) And wherever God's believing people gather in Jesus' name, the Spirit of God is there. After all, we Christians are temples of the Holy Spirit (1 Cor. 6:19) and that same Spirit Who raised Christ from the dead lives in us! (Rom. 8:11) Awesome but true! Jesus Christ, through the Holy Spirit, indwells every body in the body of Christ.

Jesus said, "I was in prison and you came to Me". (Matt.

25:36) He doesn't want His body on earth to overlook the multitudes behind bars.These men and women may also be behind spiritual bars and crying out for help.

Our church goes into an area prison - and nowhere else have we experienced such a moving of the Holy Spirit. The Lord promises, "blessed are those who hunger and thirst after righteousness, for they shall be satisfied". (Matt. 5:6) The men who come to our services are hungry for God and the Lord responds. The Holy Spirit weaves together the short teachings and testimonies as if we had pre-planned them. He may give one of us a song, another a prophecy and another a word of knowledge. It's almost breathtaking and so are the results. Often, prisoners come in droves to receive Jesus as Lord and Savior - to be born again.

The anointing (which breaks the yoke, Is.10:27) is usually strong. One night, our leader, in the back of the spartan dining room where we were meeting, saw the shekinah glory of God up front as another member of our group was teaching on building our foundation on the Rock.

One one occasion, when there was a call for the Baptism in the Holy Spirit, waves of anointing moved front to back as the great majority of men began speaking in tongues. People also get healed and delivered. Yet this move of God is featuring no one or two men or women; virtually the entire group is being used. To God alone be the glory!

Another example of Jesus using his current earthly body to bless people occurred in the same prison. A team from our Good News Church went in to conduct a service, joining a minister from another church.

From the beginning, the Holy Spirit took over. As one of the police guards led over 70 inmates in praise and worship, the very rafters seemed to ring. The anointing of God become strong. Then, in brief testimonies, one of the team spoke of Jesus not turning away from a leper. Another related how he'd faced long imprisonment but was rescued by the Lord. Another mentioned thinking of quitting a difficult situation, but getting the strength to hold on. Another told of going to church weekly, but not knowing Jesus Christ personally.

We discovered later that these testimonies spoke to different prisoners and helped them. The bottom line was 18 of the men coming forward to either receive Jesus the first time or to recommit to Him.

But, even after the service ended, the Holy Spirit kept moving. The minister from the other churh wanted prayer. His pastor had died and he was concerned about the future. As we held hands and prayed, one of our people spoke a message in tongues, another interpreted it. It was a prophetic promise and encouragement. And there was more. The minister, whom we'll call Bob, had seriously racked his arm in a motorcycle accident. As members of our team cast out the appropriate spirits, God moved. Finally, the remaining pain seemed to be gone. There was new movement in Bob's shoulder.

Someone suggested "the pelvis thing" and the Lord moved Bob's hips and he was freed further. Then someone else felt we should check his legs. One leg was about an inch shorter than the other. After the Lord grew the leg out, an arm length check showed a difference there, too. As with the leg, we took authority over a spirit of infirmity and commanded parts the back to relax and line up . The short arm grew out!.

Since in Isaiah 10:27 God tells us the anointing breaks the yoke, we can know that's exactly what happened. And, at the name of Jesus, every knee did bend, and Bob's shoulder, arms, back and legs did quite well, too.

When you and/or your family are working for God, you can expect demonic opposition, it goes with the territory. But when you're in the body of Christ, the Lord often will use your family to help.

On one recent morning at 6 AM, the Spenners received a phone call from daughter, Jenni, at Oral Roberts University. She needed prayer. It seemed that over the past few days, lumps had been appearing under her arms. They were about marble-size and the number was increasing. A visit to the doctor had elicited the comment this "could be very serious.

We'll keep our eye on this for a while." He said it could be lymphoma (a form of cancer).To Jenni, healed years earlier from lupus, the diagnosis was not exactly reassuring.

On the phone, mom and dad went into spiritual warfare. They bound fear, infirmity and other spirits. They loosed. In the name of Jesus. That was on a Wednesday morning.

The following Friday night, Jenni went to a service on campus. The message was on divine healing. The power of God was present to heal. And Jenni noticed one large lump had diminished in size.

The next morning, all of the lumps were gone. Jesus had totally healed Jenni Spenner, with assists from several parts of His body.

"Now you are Christ's body and individually members of it." (I Cor. 12:27)

An unholy quartet of losers

"No weapon that is formed against you shall prosper " (Isaiah 54:17)

Some years ago there was an American conglomerate that used the slogan, "The more you look, the more you like". Satan, our adversary, has a spiritual conglomerate of demons - the more you look, the more you don't like. Let's consider four that have been overlooked as spirits subject to us in the name of Jesus.

Stress

Take plain old everyday, everyway stress. You can observe its effects on people everywhere. In frayed nerves, frustration, irritability and the too-common inability to relax. In today's high-speed, hi-tech world, stress may be more prevalent than at any other time in history. And it's a dangerous factor in the devil's evil conglomerate. Unpleasant in itself, the spirit can open the door to a company of others, from anxiety to anger to rage to fatigue. Plus physical problems.

You mean stress is a spirit? You bet. Contrary to much we read and hear about, stress is not normal or healthy - a little or a lot of it. Just as drugs are foreign substances, so are all kinds of stress. The bottom line is if it can be cast out, there's no doubt it's a demonic spirit.

When we begin deliverance, we usually start with stress and tension (its co-worker). Most people seem to have stress and tension - even though manifestations may not constantly occur.

Not long ago, I arose early and at lunch time was very hungry, and even preparing my sandwich-type lunch, I was tense and stressed. When I told those spirits to take off, I could relax.

In the foreword, we note how a radio announcer was freed from stress, in the name of Jesus, and felt like sitting down. On another occasion a busy minister was set free from stress, then anxiety and then worry. He felt better each time - finally commenting that he was feeling much lighter.

Stress can not only uptight you, but it can cause a physical problem. In "God's Health Care Plan", we record how a young lady lost 75% of her neck and shoulder pain when stress left in Jesus' name. That's when we first realized stress was a spirit.

What's more, stress and tension can give entre to or join other spirits to affect us beyond its own capabilities. Take Jane. She wasn't feeling well and considered calling a prayer line. She definitely had been "down".

When we prayed on the phone, she was first delivered from stress and tension and noticed a difference. Anxiety also left, then confusion, followed by the ejection of a spirit of low body self image. At this point, Jane realized she was smiling. Finally she was freed from a spirit of chronic fatigue syndrome and felt even more relaxed and alert. At the end of a few minutes of God's deliverance that began with stress and tension, Jane said, "I feel great!"

These two spirits seem so prevalent that we often cast them out in our home bible fellowship meetings - with a general command. Twice, someone has seen these spirits go up through the ceiling. At Jesus' name, they must depart!

So - we don't have to be stressed out and tense; we don't have to go from stress to worse, either. Remember that Jesus said in Luke 10:19 He has given us authority over all the power of the enemy and that <u>nothing</u> shall harm us!

Chronic Fatigue Syndrome

This spirit inflicts fatigue and tiredness on a regular ba sis. You don't even have to overwork or wear yourself out, you simply are chronically fatigued.

Much has been written and discussed about this disease in this decade. It rated a cover story in a leading weekly news magazine. A lengthy book has been published. There is also, a support group for those who suffer from it. That group, National Chronic Fatigue Syndrome and Fibromyalgia Association calls CFS "the thief of vitality".

The world wishes "would there be a cure" for this energy-sapping, work-reducing and debilitating disease.

There is an answer. Cast it out in the name of Jesus like any other demonic entity.

Tim, in his fifties, is a basic member of our home bible fellowship. For over a year, he was so tired that at 5 PM he'd have to nap - at least Monday through Friday. Yet he was getting enough sleep, jogging daily and was otherwise in good health. It was frustrating. But, at one session we prayed for Tim and cast out a spirit of chronic fatigue syndrome.

Two weeks laater, he reported the daily fatigue was gone and so were the naps. Now, over four years later, Tim remains free from a spirit that's far worse than a five o'clock shadow.

Not long ago, I was praying for a lady who wanted the Lord to give her more strength. But I felt the Lord checking me and suggesting I prayed against chronic fatigue syndrome instead. When I commanded that spirit to leave,the lady felt brighter and more alert. The fatigue had lifted.

The Bible says God gives strength to His people. (Ps. 68:35) The devil would like to steal it away. He also doesn't want us to realize chronic fatigue syndrome is caused by a spirit. But when we know the truth, the Truth can set us free.

Attention Deficit Disorder

According to the National Attention Deficit Disorder Association, an estimated 3% to 15% of the U.S. population has ADD. Over 100 research studies have been published in recent years.

What is ADD? It's a neurobiological dysfunction of the brain. Afflicted people have difficulty controlling impulses, remaining focused and remembering over a long period of time. The ADDA describes this disease as "a dynamic combination of symptoms requiring treatment", genetically-transmitted , caused by a chemical imbalance or deficiency.

Let's look at it in spiritual terms. A combination of symptoms means there is more than one spirit involved. Genetically-transmitted means ADD is an inherited spirit. And the chemical imbalance indicates there is a spirit of chemical imbalance in the mix. As we give examples of deliverance that include ADD, you'll see how this can work.

To our surprise, we're finding a sizable number of people we've done deliverance on seem to have spirits of ADD as one link in a demonic chain. These people were not aware ADD was a part of their situation. And although cases of ADD alone (if there are such) have not come across our path yet, all Christians who pray deliverance should be aware of the ADD spirit and their Jesus-delegated authority over it.

For example, Philip, calling from one of the eastern states was having an itching problem which had persisted for some time. It was bothering him when he called. Notice the order of deliverance. First, we cast out a spirit of sorcery. (He had been in the occult before he became a Christian.) Then came a spirit of inherited hormonal imbalance. He felt a coolness as it departed. Since his brothers and sisters had opposed his marriage, we cast out spirits of wrath and rage. Then, since he had a problem concentrating, we loosed a spirit of attention deficit disorder. Finally, genital infirmity left. The net result - his itching had ended. ADD could have been a contributing factor, not to mention the cause of poor concentration. And - it was gone!

We picked up a clue to a possible gate of entry for this

spirit when we worked with Loretta (covered in another chapter). This lady told us, after ADD left and new peace came in, that she had much coming at her that week. There had been a death with stress, anxiety, etc along with it. If yoiu get somewhat "beside yourself" that attention problem can sneak in. A spirit of confusion also left Loretta during deliverance.

Before we finalized this book, we felt that one more major testimony would come in. And it did.

Dick's company had been out on strike a long time, and he was out of health insurance. He had physical problems including sciatica, a pinched nerve that caused back pain. Enroute to the physical freeing, we cast out a variety of emotional spirits. Three that went, in order, were dyslexia, (he had trouble reading when he was young), attention deficit disorder, inherited chemical imbalance, thyroid imbalance and metabolic imbalance. Note that ADD and inherited chemical imbalance went out in that order.

Lanny had severe pre-birth problems. His mother had labor pains at 20 weeks into her pregnancy. She was given a variety of drugs. Finally, six weeks earlier, Lanny was born. It was a difficult birth.

Years later, before he reached his teen years, Lanny had deliverance. It began with rejection (and he reported feeling much better). Among the many other spirits cast out were anger, depression, fear of breaking something, trauma, an occult curse against the family, terror, dread, stinging eyes, chronic fatigue syndrome, narcolepsy (getting sleepy at non-sleep times), and ADD/hyper.

Those weeks of pre-delivery drugs had taken their toll on the boy. But delivery by Jesus Christ had ended long years of bondage!

Bart also had pre-birth hurts. In his case, the boy's mother went into a many-weeks-early labor and drugs were necessary. He was born 12 weeks ahead of time. Then, in a neo-natal ward, Bart contracted a vicious form of spinal meningitis. Chance of recovery - 15%. A CATscan indicated his brain was black, dead. No hope.

Wrong. A prayer chain went into action - and so did God. The boy was miraculously healed. He was called Mt. Sinai's "miracle" baby.

Years later, not yet ten, deliverance came to Bart. He was freed from asthma and ear problems. (The heat of the Holy Spirit came into his ears through hands on ministry that included commands to spirits.) A spirit of chronic fatigue syndrome left the boy.

Then came the big one. In the name of Jesus, Attention Deficit Disorder was cast out- and he felt it. One result of this demonic disease had been trouble concentrating. Unshackled, Bart was free from ADD!

Low Body Self Image

Judy had a weight problem (not exactly uncommon in our rich-foods part of the world). In the course of commanding prayer, we cast out a spirit of low body self image - and she said she wanted to laugh. Something had lifted from her.

Low body self image - we're finding it's been bugging a lot of people. Not just because of obesity, either. It could be perceived appearance, something someone once said - a variety of reasons. But, when we take the thought of it, instead of taking that thought captive (2 Cor.10:5), we may also take in the spirit.

God doesn't want us to put ourselves down. He made us and we're precious in His sight. Real humility is seeing things as He does. When we don't, the devil can successfully lie to us and get two strikes on us before we even get up to bat.

Isn't it comforting to know that such debilitators as stress & tension, chronic fatigue syndrome, attention deficit disorder and low body self image are subject to the name of Jesus - and, in His name, those demons are subject to us!

Five categories of demons

"Truly, I say to you, whoever says to this mountain,'Be taken up and cast into the sea' and does not doubt in his heart, but believes what he says is going to happen, it shall be granted him." (Mark 11:23)

Notice Jesus tells us to speak to THIS mountain - be specific. The longer we minister, the more we realize the most effective way to cast out a spirit is to address the specific spirit by name. If someone has a problem with timidity, don't speak to fear (although that's often around as well), but speak to timidity.

You may ask why not simply command, "Come out of him, you foul spirit"! There are two reasons for normally not doing that. First, it may not work. When I was in the army and they called Bill out of line, I didn't go. In deliverance, on one occasion, for example, we spoke to fear and nothing happened, but when we addressed fear of rejection, that spirit left. Second, and very important, unless there is a manifestation of a SPECIFIC spirit leaving, you and the deliveree won't know what left and has to be defended against later. Maybe there was a spirit of anger involved, but if it leaves after a general command, no one may know it was included.

Doesn't everyone with an anger problem know it? No. Once we dealt with someone who had anger. Everyone else saw it, but the person involved couldn't see it. That spirit, or another one, had blocked recognition. I had fear for many years, but couldn't see it until a time of deliverance, when it manifested unmistakeably.

Whenever you can, use a rifle instead of a shotgun. Be a sharpshooter. Hit the bullseye!

When we were praying for Lenora, nothing happened when

we spoke to self-rejection. But, there was noticeable deliverance from rejection and fear of rejection. Gwen had no reaction to despair, but she reacted strongly when grief was addressed. Freda, after death in the family, was very down. Finally, pinpointing a spirit of sadness brought tears and release. And so on.

What follows is one of the main reasons we're writing this book - to pass on what we've learned in the arena of pinpoint deliverance.

There may not be just one kind of spirit of fear, anger or anything else. Chronologically alone, there can be at least five categories of each.

PRENATAL SPIRITS

The Bible recounts in John 1:1 that the Word (Jesus) was in the beginning. Unfortunately, too often the word not of God can affect an unborn child. We're told that a baby in the womb can hear and understand from the age of about four months. And words, from mom, dad, brother, sister, nurse, anyone can have a profound effect on that child and open a door for one or more evil spirits to enter that innocent and helpless baby. A spirit that enters before birth can logically be labeled a prenatal spirit. And it can affect that individual throughout life.

There is someone we'll call Tess who has had some difficulty fitting in, feeling comfortable with other people. It began in the womb; words had been spoken, and she didn't want to be born. How was this prenatal situation discovered years later? A word of knowledge from God. However, it isn't usually necessary, as we've demonstrated earlier, to have a word of knowledge. A history of parental bickering or the knowledge a child wasn't wanted, can flag the possibility of a prenatal spirit of anger, resentment, rejection, fear of rejection, self-rejection, etc. In the case of adoption, though, there is usually no knowledge of parental background. The comments of natural parents who may not have wanted the child could have affected it in the womb.

Camille had been rejected before she was born - and she knew it before she was born. Through much of her life, there had been difficulties with close relatives. During deliverance, there was a definite manifestation of the departure of the spirit of prenatal rejection. Children unwanted before birth can feel unwanted long after birth. Unless there is a deliverance, that spirit can remain and cause damage.

Dede's life wasn't as pleasant as it should have been. No wonder. She needed, and received, deliverance from spirits of pride, anger, hate and fear. Plus one that could have opened the door for the others - a spirit of prenatal rejection. When you've been rejected before you've even seen the light of day, you can wall yourself with pride, be angry, hate people and fear them.

It's no secret that when mom is into drug abuse, her unborn child can be affected. Ask a teacher of learning disability kids. She'll tell you it's often the case.

CHILDHOOD SPIRITS

Lydia had head pain. When a spirit of prenatal ADD (Attention Deficit Disorder) was commanded out, most of the pain left. When childhood ADD was cast out, the remainder of the pain left. Gus had been an alcoholic. During deliverance, he not only lost a spirit of inadequacy, but also a spirit of childhood inadequacy.

Elsewhere in this book, you can read of a man who picked up a childhood spirit of alcoholism by considerable drinking that began at age 14. Around that same age, a childhood spirit of pornography entered a boy (now an adult) when he started looking at pornography brought into the home. Both felt relief in these areas during deliverance.

It may seem almost unbelievable, but at one session, we cast out over 25 different childhood spirits from one person. Among them were childhood terror, fear of violence, trauma, rebellion, self-pity, anger, insecurity, frustration, sadness, rejection and fear of rape. Getting free, primarily from childhood spirits, brought improvement emotionally and physically.

INHERITED SPIRITS

In Numbers 14:18 we read that God visits the iniquity of the fathers on the children to third and fourth generations. It may not be our fault, but we can be affected by a generational or inherited spirit from generations back.

Way back in Genesis, the devil was cursing families. Cain (Gen. 4:8) killed his brother Abel. That spirit of murder continued down the family line. In Genesis 4:23, one of Cain's descendants, Lamach, boasted, "I have killed a man for wounding me; and a boy striking me"! That inherited murder spirit was strong on him. Have things changed nearly 6000 years later? Not much. The big change came with the Lord Jesus Christ, who defeated the devil and his kingdom. Now, we, His followers, have been given authority over all the power of the enemy. That baalish buck can stop with us!

Consider Rita Hunt. When we were interviewing with Rev. Jeff Melvin on WWWG, a tell-it-like-it-is Christian station in Rochester, NY, Rita called in to mention her remarkable healing and deliverance. Later, we called her and heard the following story:

In 1994, Rita became quite ill. She vomited daily and was losing weight. Her shoulder-length hair was falling out. Testing plus a biopsy indicated a serious problem. The blood test ran T-4 and a high TSH. Those swollen glands and other symptoms were caused by a goiter. She was either borderline hypothyroid or borderline hyperthyroid. Either way, Rita was a very sick lady. She needed a 12-week leave from work.

The thyroid problem ran in the family. Her mother's thyroid gland had been removed a year earlier. Her aunt (who had passed away) lost her thyroid three years before the spirit hit Rita.

Rita called her mother for a prayer of agreement that God had healed her. Others prayed. Rita cried out to God. She told Him, "I know I'm healed", and "I have to believe you for myself". She knew she couldn't rely on the faith of her pastor husband.

She did something else. Rita, and others, broke that generational curse, speaking to it in the name of Jesus Christ, the name above all names.

What happened? Rita's appetite came back. Food stayed down. Her hair started growing back. And the swelling began to recede. Her energy level was up - and she kept thanking God and speaking healing scriptures.

A year from the first biopsy, another was taken, plus blood testing. The indicators were down, the biopsy was negative. The honest doctor commented, "I don't understand" But Rita understood. In the name of Jesus, she had driven off that inherited spirit and the healing she sought and claimed had come to pass.

In the autumn of 1996, Rita was enjoying more than Indian Summer. She was basking in the God of her salvation!

Oh, yes. Before Rita took her 12-week leave for sickness, she spotted another lady in the office reading "God Heals Today", our book which chronicles over 70 medically-confirmed cases of divine healing. The lady gave it to her. And Rita says what she read helped her. More proof that Jesus Christ, who took our sicknesses and pains, (Is. 53:14) is no respecter of persons. (Acts 10:34). What He'll do for one, He'll do for another!

Look at the group of inherited spirits that Stanley was cursed with. Fear, timidity, inadequacy and fear of it, self-belittlement, hatred of women, fear of verbal abuse, self-doubt and self-recrimination. With losers like that passed down to you, it's not easy to be a winner in life. But, deliverance is making a difference. And rebuking any of those enemies that try to return will help him walk more confidently and successfully!

Trina had overcome alcoholism. Her marriage was secure. Yet she could feel more secure. She had known rejection, distress, depression, sadness and confusion. All of those spirits were loosed from her. But - the first to leave was an inherited spirit of fear of dementia - losing her mind. Imagine having that one around and the freedom that came when it left!

RESIDUAL SPIRITS

Dottie's mariage was rocky. During deliverance, many of her besiegers had to go. Of all of the departures, perhaps the most important was that of a residual spirit of doubt. It left through a big yawn. Doubt is the opposite of faith. Without faith, Hebrews 11:6 reveals, it's impossible to please God. That kind of spirit can also be a strong deterrent to relationships of trust within a family.

How do we define a residual spirit? One that's been residing in someone a long time. One lady had been suffering pain on and off for over ten years. There was no relief until a residual spirit of pain was driven off. Then she was freed after all those years. But, speaking to pain didn't help, it had to be the residual spirit - a long time tenant.

We've discussed and chronicled prenatal, inherited, childhood and residual spirits. What's the fifth category? Just what most of us have been accustomed to driving out, the plain no-time-period spirit. For example, take rejection.There are prenatal, inherited, childhood, residual spirits - plus simply the spirit of rejection. Casting out the latter may do it. Yet a person could also have other categories. Check it out. You may be surprised at what you discover!

As I was writing this book, I had an opportunity to pray for a busy man who had blurred vision. An object he held at arm's length wasn't clear. After casting out tension, stress, anxiety and a few other spirits, I went after blindness, ocular infirmity and blurriness or cloudiness. He reported his sight was improved - going in and out; now clear, now blurry.

Irritated at the devil's games, I angrily commanded inherited, childhood, prenatal and residual spirits to leave him, in the name of Jesus Christ. This made a pronounced difference. He reported his sight was "much better". It was no longer varying. He could hold an object at arm's length and see it clearly.

By addressing the spectrum of specific spirits - prenatal, childhood, residual, inherited (and probably just the plain name), I must have included the precise culprit or culprits. And that's what it took for the Holy Spirit to do the work!

Spirits can come into one's life anywhere along the way - from pre-birth (another proof God considers a child in the womb to be a person - and the devil does,too!) However, they can also be forced out in the name of Jesus anywhere along the way!

Light on new areas for victory

"we are not ignorant of his (the devil's) devices" (II Cor. 2:11 KJV)

Since we completed "God's Health Care Plan" two years ago, we've come across a coven of evil spirits we didn't know existed. We feel it's important to share what we've learned with you.

As you read this book, you will find references to imbalance spirits more than 25 times. We've been encountering - and casting them out - often.

God's revelation began well over a year ago when we were praying for two people (mother and son) who were perspiring inordinately. As we prayed in the spirit, He gave us the words, "chemical imbalance". Accordingly, we cast out such spirits from both persons. With the son, we included inherited chemical imbalance.

About two weeks later, the mother reported her excess perspiring had ended. The son's situation was improved.

It's a known fact that a chemical imbalance in the body can affect the brain. Imagine, if you will, the possible effects of a biochemical imbalance, a thyroid imbalance, a metabolic imbalance, a hormonal imbalance, a sugar imbalance, etc. Also imagine how such imbalances can be inherited and adversely affect generations.

In Chapter 15, you'll read about a middle-aged man whohad physical problems that included ADD and dyslexia. When we cast it out along with other spirits which included ADD, inherited chemical imbalance, thyroid imblance and metabolic imbalance , there was a notable improvement.

17. Imbalance Spirits

In Chapter 14, we recount the case of a young man who had been taking enzymes for digestive problems. Here, again, God gave a word of knowledge - "chemical imbalance". When that spirit was commanded out in Jesus' name, he felt something lift and leave. Spirits of biochemical imbalance, hormonal imbalance and metabolic imbalance were also driven out. And the young man felt a new peace. Those spirits had entered and thrown him out of balance.

Art told his doctor's nurse, "I feel better than I have in a year!" Why? Look at the record. In 1989, his stomach hemorraghed because of a recurring ulcer. He had suffered almost continuing stomach pain. Then in 1995, he started taking medication for the pain.

Among the spirits he lost one night at a home meeting were blood pressure imbalance (his blood pressure rose and fell according to his emotions), chemical imbalance (we spoke to "inherited, residual or otherwise') and metabolic imbalance. At the end of the meeting, most of the pain was gone.

Ronnie still had side effects from an accident 15 years earlier. Working regularly was difficult. Fortunately his mental capabilities continued to return. One of the spirits that he was freed from was hormonal imbalance.

A lady, noted in Chapter 7, had a history of high blood pressure that came on from time to time. Resultantly, we cast out a spirit of blood pressure imbalance. This was one in the chain of spirits that contributed to a severe headache.

In that same chapter, someone with breathing problems had further improvement as soon as thyroid and hormonal imbalance were commanded to leave.

In Chapter 19, an unfortunate woman put up with years of menopausal bleeding. She was helped with the logical expulsion of a spirit of estrogen imbalance.

Yetta was under heavy pressure. Holding up, she was near buckling. That night she lost many emotional spirits -

plus all of what we call the core imbalance group - chemical, biochemical, thyroid, metabolic and hormonal. A body out of balance gives you less to fight with.

Pamela struggled with infertility - also PMS. She lost spirits of thyroid and metabolic imbalance. Ask her if there are such things as imbalance spirits!

A woman in her forties had been diagnosed with hormone imbalance, hormone fluctuation and menopause. To understate, it was a bother. Telephone deliverance covered other territory also. However - when we cast out a spirit of estrogen imbalance, she felt the heat and power of the Holy Spirit come on her body. No question of what happened. Farewell, estrogen imbalance!

On it goes. If you think you or someone you care about may have any imbalances, check the testimonies in the book. Start with the index. Medical science is discovering more about imbalance effects. One (non-medical) ad states chemical imblance is a cause of overweight. Could be. These spirits have been affecting people for too long. The time has come to get rid of them - and the problems they cause!

Chemical, biochemical, thyroid, metabolic, hormonal, blood pressure, estrogen, sugar - and more. They are demonic enemies - but like any others, they must go at the name of Jesus Christ. He wants us to be in perfect balance!

Identification allows ejection

"But you, brethren, are not in darkness" (I Thess. 5:4)

Jesus is the light of the world and His Holy Spirit wants to enlighten us in every area, including spiritual warfare. Today, He's showing the body of Christ more and more of the spirits that have too long remained incognito.

One Christian we know wanted to cut down on his secular televiewing. It wasn't easy. But, after we cast out a spirit of TV addiction and one of TV craving, he noticed a difference.

A long-time Christian craved foods she was better off without or foods she could eat in smaller quantities. Sometimes this desire was uncontrollable - a sure sign of demonic control. Then, when a spirit of sugar craving was expelled, she was aware of a difference.

Sound off the wall? Jesus said, by their fruits we would know them. (Matt. 7:16) Notice the evil fruit and notify the evil spirit to get out. Expel it by speaking to it by the name of what it causes: anger, resentment, self-pity, lying, swearing and so on.

We were doing deliverance one afternoon. The lady before Faye and I was subject to migraine headaches. Knowing the spirits are subject to us (Luke 10:17) we commanded the migraine offender to leave. Nothing transpired. Then, through a word of knowledge, we learned of lobol migraine. When we cast it out, the lady's head became clear.

There are spirits of trauma. And since so many people have had traumatic experiences somewhere along the way, this understanding can prove quite helpful. One lady reacted when we cast out pre-natal and then post-natal trauma. She'd had such a spirit on each side of the birth canal. Additionally, she lost spirits of trauma-fear and trauma-terror. A key spirit in the deliverance of another woman was verbal-abuse trauma. How relatively common this type of oppression is for children growing up and husbands and wives.

A pair of spirits that can go together are abandonment and fear of it. We've come across these more than once. The abandonment doesn't have to be a life-threatening situation, either. It can simply be a child getting separated from mom or dad in a supermarket. One of our granddaughters was temporarily "lost" from grandma at our church's hallelujah (instead of halloween) party. A few days later, she didn't want to go to preschool, fearing grandmother wouldn't be right there with her. And this is a very outgoing child.

Here's an interesting and logical group of spirits that could be afflicting more individuals and families than you might expect. Taylor is a very capable mother. Yet her family background affected her in the here and now. She had an outlook problem with money - didn't really expect to prosper. She was prone to squeeze what she had. And this was not a single mom. She worked and so did her husband.

Taylor was delivered from spirits of inherited poverty, inherited lack, frugality and love of money. (You don't have to have it to love it!) In fact, there was a strong manifestation on the loss of that last one. Since the love of money is "the root of all kinds of evil" (1 Tim. 6:10), the spirit can be a door-opener to a host of other spirits. Some people pinch pennies. It's one thing to be a good steward and another to be overly frugal. Yes, there is a spirit of frugality!

The Lord doesn't want us sad; He wants us joyful. After all, the joy of the Lord is our strength. (Neh. 8:10) One lady had a death in the family and a key to getting over it was the expulsion of a spirit of sadness. We've found this demon is fairly common and likes to take the joy out of life.

One evening, we expelled a spirit of deep hurt from someone being ministered to and someone else in the room was also set free.

Verbal abuse is not only an action, it's also a spirit. Crying was a manifestation when this one left a lady who had put up with it a long time.

A spirit of household compliance? In a deliverance session, one of those present received a word of knowledge. When the spirit was cast out, there was a strong manifestation. The person freed had been displaying something in her home that God considers an idol. Because she was trying to please one or more people, the Christian lady of the house was giving entre to a demon.

The fear category has many faces. One of them we've encountered more than once is a spirit of fear of mother dying. This spirit helps preclude trusting God for the future. Wonderful as mothers are, God is our source. Particularly in the case of adults, this kind of apprehension is inordinate and can prove emotionally sapping.

Another face of fear is the fear of success. In my own career in advertising, I would seem to reach a certain level and not be able to break through beyond it. A spirit of inadequacy and the fear of inadequacy can ally with the fear of success and keep us from reaching the position God is calling us to.

Mental torment can be overwhelming and can be caused by a spirit with that name. It can come from a spirit of fear (a very common enemy). God does warn us in 1 John 4:18 that fear has torment. (KJV) And since fear is a sin, it paves the way for that vicious mental torment.

Depression alone is oppressive, but it can also lead to spirits of despondency and despair. The next intruder can then be a spirit of suicide. The devil's five step plan for self destruction includes discouragement, depression, despondency, despair and finally suicide. It's a dangerous downhill cycle. We have, quite a few times, cast out both despondency and despair, following depression.Those mullygrubs can get you down - and out.

Ever know someone who was indecisive? Couldn't make up his or her mind? That state of mind can prevent fruitful decisions and cause anguish. The root could be a spirit of indecision. Fear or fear of success, fear of failure and the futaure, plus inadequacy can open the door. Who needs any of them?

Doreen was having pain in her bones. We discovered it was caused by a group of spirits. These included bone calcification, calcification, disc infirmity and (in this case) both rheumatoid and osteoarthritis. With that lineup, you'd hurt, too. But when these and other spirits were cast out, their game was over. And, Doreen felt much better.

Maxine had finally separated from her husband. The marriage had lasted for years and it was an unhappy one. In the aftermath, she was attacked by many spiritual enemies. In the name of Jesus, she lost many spirits, pre and post-separation.

But, for Maxine to know even greater relief and freedom, there was one more spirit to go. Through the years, she had leaned on and depended on her husband. He made the important decisions, she went along.

Learning this, we addressed a spirit we had never cast out before - a spirit of co-dependency. And it left, Marcia had a powerful manifestation.

So - even the much-discussed problem of co-dependency is demonic. Like any other spirit, it must go in the name of Jesus Christ!

Winston Churchill was no scholastic giant. His grades in school ran around the C level. Maybe no instructor challenged him. (Later, of course, he was greatly challenged and rose to that challenge to provide leadership to save England - and perhaps the entire free world - in World War II)

Maybe young Winston was bored. Uninterested. Could

have been.

Well, he certainly wasn't the only one to drift uninterestedly through classes. Take Frankie. He was bored. Couldn't seem to want to get involved in classwork. His mind wandered off.

However, during a deliverance session, Frankie and we were surprised. One of the spirits we spoke to was boredom. And he had a definite reaction. God had freed the young man from a spirit of boredom. Hopefully, he'll get with it in future classes.

The devil wants us bored - to miss out. To lose out, in every way possible. Even with boredom.

In how many marriages is there a problem in the bedroom? One partner frustrated because the other seems to be holding back, seems inhibited? Probably more than we'll ever know. The devil hates marriage and doesn't want husbands and wives to enjoy rightful physical pleasure.

If you fall into that category, rejoice! Your deliverance ccould be at hand. During a deliverance session in Mid-America, a lady was set free. Which means her husband should benefit as well. She, with a strong manifestation, lost a spirit of sexual inhibition. The spirit was inherited, generational, passed down from mother and perhaps even farther back. Other spirits were involved, but with sexual inhibition out, this lady can get on with an even happier marriage!

You name it, the devil's got it. These are specific spirits and they must go when addressed by name. We've only mentioned a few of the spirits you might not be aware of or consider. The more we minister, the more we encounter.

Even if it seems to sound silly, such as a *spirit of blossom* (mentioned in another chapter) try it; you might be pleasantly surprised. Ignorance is not bliss. It's one of Satan's shields!

Dismantlement of the domain of darkness

"Nay, in all these things
we are more than conquerors
through him that loved us ."
(Romans 8:37 KJV)

Jesus makes it clear in Mark 16 that all believers should be casting out demons. In Luke 10:19, He says we have authority over all the power of the enemy. And in that chapter, He rejoiced greatly in the Spirit because His followers discovered that, in His name, demons were subject to them. That still holds. I believe the Lord still rejoices when the enemy is driven off and people are set free. So, let's be glad and decide to go and do likewise as we look over marvels God is doing today.

Tumors

Growths, internal and external, are infernal. The Lord, of course, is able to deal with any and all of them.

When Vince De John was still a Chicago banker, he was ministering to people. In respsonse to a phone call, Vince visited a home to pray for man with a cap on. When the Christian banker arrived, the man removed his cap. On his head were two large, black tumors. Doctors were concerned because the growing tumors were approaching the brain.

Vince taught the man briefly on divine healing. Just a week earlier, he had felt impressed to study the subject. After doing this preparatory work, Vince rebuked the tumors and commanded them to be gone, in the name of Jesus. Then, everyone in the room prayed in agreement for the healing.

Two weeks later, the man awoke to discover both tumors were no longer implanted in his head, but resting on his pillow. The Lord had done what He promises in His word - and healed - bringing a frightening event to a fear-free happy ending.

Sometimes you don't know the full or lasting result of commanding prayer at the time you pray. Mona had pains in her legs and areas of her back for many years. There was weakness as well. Managing stairs was no fun. She'd been harassed too long. And nothing seemed to end it.

One day, Faye and I prayed for her. We spoke to a variety of spirits, including sciatica, pain, inflammation and several others. There was immediate improvement.

But, it wasn't until many weeks later we heard the final results. The problem had been eliminated - and Mona continued to be free from it.

"Free" does seem to be an appropriate word for people who've been putting up with infirmity and then get unshackled. After all, Jesus said in the Fourth Chapter of Luke that He came to set the captives free. That included Mona - and it can include you and those you can help!

Letitia isn't one to complain. But she had good reason to. Consider the torment of many years of insomnia, menopausal bleeding, tiring easily and general weakness, plus long-term back pain.

Jesus Christ, the same yesterday, today and forever, has already borne all of the above junk. So, it didn't have to be Letitia's arsenic cup of tea.

In about an hour and a quarter, ministering Christians were able to help the Lord change things for the better. The lightening of the load and lifting of the burden began with the expulsion of a spirit of chronic fatigue syndrome. Then estrogen imbalance was cast out. Residual frustration had to go. A spirit of weakness departed, followed by immune system infirmity. The back pain left when a spirit of inherited arthritis did. Letitia felt the heat of the Holy Spirit when she laid hands on herself and other Christians cast out a spirit of candida (that yeast infection that can rise up and spoil a person). A spirit of unrest left next. A driving spirit took off and the manifestation was marked, with the heat of the Lord again coming on Letitia. The same strong manifestation was evident with the expulsion of spirits of underactive thyroid and low blood pressure.

Letitia felt better. She was pleased to know those long-term enemies weren't around any more!

Why did the session take over an hour? Often, to get an understanding and where they're coming from, you have to talk with people. Counselors know this and co-deliverers with Christ should also be aware of it.,

Co-dependency

When someone is overly dependent on someone else, it's unhealthy. It's also a spirit. Casting it out sets people free.

Meg called late at night. She had just returned home from the office - and barely made it. Weak and dizzy, with pressure in her head, she prayed hard to drive safely to her new residence.

Her marriage had recently come apart and Meg had moved. Now she was driving herself to work harder and better - and longer. This had been close to an eleven-hour day. She had eaten nearly nothing in 24 hours, which didn't help. But when a marriage of more than ten years finally dissipates, what she felt and did is understandable.

Meg's deliverance began with tension and stress and then anxiety (a major stronghold). She felt more calm. Then fear was commanded out. When rejection left, she reported feeling more peace. Self-rejection followed. (When a marriage fails , no matter whose fault, there can be self putdown.) Now tension in her forehead was gone. The next spirit successfully addressed was discouragement; inadequacy was next to go. As we spoke to a spirit of trauma, a headache suddenly manifested. But, when childhood trauma was dispatched, the headache left. The next step - driving out a spirit of worry.

Then, the Lord gave a breakthrough word of knowledge - co-dependency. We commanded it to go and Meg experienced a powerful release. In her long and unhappy marriage, she had become heavily dependent on her husband, a major reason why she had held on, miserable, through the years. Now - she was set free from that spirit!

Continuing, we cast out hormonal imbalance, and Meg was even more peaceful. Next, we attacked the physical trespassers. She had a family history of sinus problems. So we cast out sinusitis, allergic rhinitis, catarrh, post-nasal drip and bronchitis (inherited, allergic or otherwise). And pressure left Meg's head, Finally, we commanded fatigue and dizziness to go. Then she was able to focus clearly.

Faye now dictated the list of expelled spirits (in order) and advised Meg to stand against them daily. Meg was a happy lady after that hour-and-a-half deliverance. Jesus, by the Holy Spirit, did it, when we commanded the spirits to leave in His mighty, overcoming name.

In 1995, Jack had an almost incredible healing. Since shortly after birth, he had no fingernails. Then, one day in church, a variety of prayer, including hands-on and commanding in the name of Jesus, brought a miracle. Over a period of weeks, fingernails grew in to cover close to 50% of the appropriate areas on Jack's fingers.

In 1996, Jack came to church crippled with a sore and swollen foot. He couldn't wear a shoe. In a work accident, his foot became wedged, as I recall, under a forklift. The foot was extremely bruised, a large blister had broken, there was the possibility of infection and walking was very painful. His skin had been sensitive since birth because of epidermilosis bolsis.

Knowing Jack also had emotional problems, we began there. We cast out tension, anxiety and frustration. Then, we laid hands on the injured foot and commanded spirits of infirmity, swelling, inflammation and pain to leave. To no avail.

Talking to Jack, we discovered some information and returned to work.The following spirits were ejected in Jesus' name: Kali (Jack worked with Hindus and Kali is an Indian"goddess".), trauma, and we prayed for healing of emotions (great emotion then seemed to well up in him), baal, and ashteroth (pagan "deities"). Somewhere around this time, Jack realized the foot pain was gone. Epidermal deficiency was addressed. Then, inherited alcoholism left, followed by religion, tradition and idolatry plus inherited mariolatry.

When he was younger, Jack had played with an ouija board, so that spirit was ejected. We dispatched pharmakia (he had been on just about all drugs except heroin). Now, Jack felt and looked better. He could walk on the injured foot without pain - even bend it.

When we next saw Jack, he reported his foot was fine. It was definitely healed. As God's word says in Philippians 2:10, at the name of Jesus, every knee should bend. And that also includes every foot!

Jim Powell is one of the many nice guys among the Christian broadcasters. After we interviewed on his station in Alabama, we were able to pray for him. He had both Type Two Diabetes and a prostate problem.

To begin with, we cast out those common robbers; stress and tension. A few other common spirits were eliminated. Then, in the name of Jesus, we commanded diabetes spirits to leave. By the time the brief session was over, Jim felt better.

Talking to him many weeks later, we discovered all of the symptoms of the prostate ailment had disappeared. The diabetes was still around. After praying against inherited spirits of chemical imbalance, bio-chemical imbalance, thyroid imbalance, metabolic imbalance, hormonal imbalance and sugar imbalance, Jim felt a reaction with each departure. Then we commanded the inherited diabetes to leave. We're waiting to hear the happy results.

This is the success story of Jeanne Ann, taken from her own handwritten testimony and attested to by her pastor of

Word of Life Church in Elk Grove Village, a Chicago suburb.

In March of 1995, Jeanne Ann went up for prayer at her church. She had unhealthy lungs and ribs. Her ribs were "so stuck", so immobile, that her lungs were prevented from expanding and her diaphragm from dropping. Air could enter only small pockets concentrated below the rib cage. Her lung capacity was dimunitive.

Pastor Vince De John commanded her rib cage to become normal in the name of Jesus. Jeanne Ann felt her left arm, which was bent, being pulled down to her ribs. The next day, she visited her physical therapist. This time, when she took a deep breath, her ribs moved laterally. She had more lung capacity - her lungs could expand.

Here's part two of her testimony, eleven months later, Jeanne Ann experienced sharp pain in her left leg. This time, she didn't need any outside help. She had learned her authority in the name of Jesus Christ. When she commanded the pain to leave in His name, it left immediately. Then a spirit of depression was commanded out and that lifted instantaneously. Jeanne Ann had been well taught. No longer would she have to suffer because of a lack of knowledge!

Hearing

Monaural hearing for 17 years is not God's highest and best. But when Ricky became a Christian at age 2l, he had been without hearing in his left ear since he was four.

Ricky had come to the right place. The ministering evangelist commanded the deaf spirits to leave the young man in the name of Jesus Christ. Suddenly, Ricky could hear through his left ear, and the stereo equipment God had given him at birth was putting out properly. The Lord had restored his full hearing and gave him new confidence for functioning effectively in the world around him!

Sight

It was a church service in the Canadian province of Maniatoba, on an Indian reservation. A boy, six at the time, was born blind. In the beginning of his school years, he - and his parents - would learn a lesson they would never forget.

The boy was brought forward for prayer. The evangelist prayed for him with the authority Jesus gives His believers. The spirit of blindness was commanded to leave. And - instantly - the blind eye opened. The boy, for the first time in his life, had sight in both eyes.

In Boston, another six-year-old boy was blind in one eye. The devil had robbed of half his sight. But God was on the scene, and when Ray Martin was ministering, he commanded blind spirits to leave in the name of Jesus. Immediately, God restored sight to the boy - and a new infilling of faith to those at the meeting. Jesus still opens blind eyes!

Insanity

The scene, once more, is Canada.This time, British Columbia. On stage, another showdown between Jesus Christ and Satan.

Mara was out of her mind. She tried to rip the shirt off the visiting evangelist. The man of God commanded the devil out of her in the name of Jesus. The indwelling demons threw her to the floor. It took six women to hold her down. Her eyes rolled; they seemed to protrude.

A demon in Mara spoke the words, “I want my momma!” Then Mara spit in her mother’s face and declared, “I hate you!” Meanwhile the evangelist kept commanding the demons to leave in the name of Jesus. In minutes, the abusing spirits were cast out of Mara. Her body relaxed - she was free from that infestation.

Now in her right mind, Mara accepted Jesus Christ as her Lord and was also baptized in the Holy Spirit. As the Fifth Chapter of Corinthians II states, old things had passed away, all things had become new. New sanity. New birth. New infilling with the Holy Spirit. And a new future for a young lady whom God loves very much.

Drugs

Jeremy became hooked on drugs late in high school. Then, he graduated from lesser stuff to cocaine. For most of the next 16 years, he was an addicted user.

Then, at 33, he received Jesus Christ into his heart. With Christian help, drug and other spirits were cast out of the young man who "couldn't stop" his heroin and cocaine habit. "I felt the power of God all over me", Jeremy remembers. And, in the name of Jesus, he was delivered.

Today, at 42, Jeremy walks free from drugs. He's happily married and a loving husband and father. Buat he hasn't forgotten where here he came from, so he helps at a treatment center for others leaving the drug scene.

How does Jeremy stay free? He knows his authority in Jesus Christ. And, he's constantly renewing his mind with the word of God. The truth set him free and that's what keeps him free!

Alcoholism

Rob's telephone deliverance was in depth, yet lasted only about 45 minutes.

He, as his father, had been an alcoholic., One night, this young Christian went to his knees and cried out to Jesus to take his drinking obsession from him. The next morning, he awoke with no desire to drink. He didn't touch a drop for the next four years.

Then, he fell, and returned to drinking. Why? For three years, he worked with abused children and became emotionally and physically drained. Exhausted, he became depressed and sought escape in his old habit. In addition, he suffered from gastritis, reflux disease (fluid in the esophogus rose instead of dropped), irritable bowel syndrome and hiatal hernia.

Here's the order of deliverance: anxiety, fear, alcohol, rejection and fear of rejection (his family and others rejected him, inherited self-rejection, inherited control and power and inadequacy. Next came two childhood spirits - childhood inadequacy and childhood fear of inadequacy. Then, carrying on in the name of Jesus, we drove out discouragement, inherited chemical imbalance (through a word of knowledge), inherited biochemical imbalance, inherited metabolic imbalance --then a loud noise blanketed telephone communication. He hung up and re-called.

Freedom fighting continued with hormonal imbalance. Since Rob had difficulty concentrating, inherited ADD was cast out. Chronic fatigue syndrome left next. Discovering he had been diagnosed with obsessive compulsive behavior, we dispatched a spirit of obsessive compulsion. Residual anger and rage left. Suicide was also successfully driven out. (The spirit entered even though he had vowed never to kill himself.) Legalism, low body self image and trauma were cast out (He had witnessed someone sexually abuse a friend). Fear of intimacy left , then - residual alcoholism and childhood alcoholism , (he began drinking at 14), ended the emotional deliverance.

At the conclusion of his deliverance, Rob was a happier man. He felt better and you could hear it in his voice. We gave him the list of ejected spirits to stand against daily.

The spirits that came on him at 14 were key to setting him free. Childhood trauma can affect a person for a lifetime. Unless we allow God to do something about it.

Incest/Rape

There can be a shade of difference. Darkness, either way.

Annette had been told of in-family sexual abuse of her. She already had prayer for sinus problems. But the long-festering problem remained. Did Annette remember the incest? She may have subconsciously blocked the memory. But Jesus wanted to release her.

When a spirit of deep abuse trauma was cast out, she felt more calm. Guilt and shame were two of other spirits that followed. Fear of past rape and self-condemnation also left. Inherited anger was driven out. These were vital and reflected the past.

When the deliverance ended, there was a deep peace on Annette and in the room. Months later, she reported she was functioning better and more confidently with friends and family. And, she's a happier person!

Abuse/Trauma

Sean is an increasingly successful businessman. On his way up. However, his past hurts were making waves in his family. Growing up, Sean had been abused - physically, emotionally and mentally. That he has done so well, speaks well of the man. But - the end of those inherited barnacles was at hand.

A Christian knowledgeable in deliverance took authority in the name of Jesus. Inherited spirits of trauma in all three categories were cast out - with hands on Sean's chest.

The power of God came in and there was a definite release. The praying Christian asked God to heal the residue from those old hurts.

Now, Sean has even more freedom to press on to his "upward call of God in Christ Jesus". (Phil. 3:14)

After church one Sunday, Benny wanted prayer for a staph infection. A fellow Christian offered to pray and laid a hand on Benny's chest. Benny then told him the chest was where the infection resided. Then, his praying brother commanded a spirit of staphylococcus and other pertinent spirits to leave in the name of Jesus.

Benny commented that even though his friend felt cold on the surface, it felt like an electric blanket in his body.

Less than a week later, Benny divulged the sores caused by the staph infection were mostly gone. After more hands-on prayer, he reported he was free from the remaining sores and itching. Only some scabs remained. His Father had healed Benny through commanding prayer and ministry in the name of His victorious Son!

I had just completed a phone interview on "God's Health Care Plan", when the Lord set up a demonstration. An engineer-announcer had, for about two years, surface cuts on his fingers. From time to time, his hands would hurt . The situation was not only painful and unsightly, but a bother to an engineer who used his hands often at the station.

First, stress, tension and anxiety were cast out and he noticed a difference. Then, spirits of cuts, inflammation, etc. we're commanded to leave in Jesus' name. He felt the evidence of God moving on the hand that wasn't holding the phone. God was healing him. Since Jesus paid for those cuts, why should His brother pay for them?

AIDS/HIV

The disease we weren't even aware of 25 years ago has become a major plague in America and elsewhere. We believe that AIDS and HIV Positive are both spirits. In praying for people so afflicted, we haven't known definite healings, but many we've prayed for have felt the power of God when we commanded those spirits to leave them. Often, when we took authority in Jesus' name, these hurting people knew something happened. Often, it has been "in my head" where there was a noted reaction. We haven't followed up, but feel God was healing. Unfortunately, most Christians don't know how to stand against diseases and may get afflicted or reafflicted.

On the phone, we prayed for a man whok was not a homosexual but somehow had become HIV Positive. We spoke to spirits of AIDS and HIV Positive and he felt a tingling on his body. Then, in Jesus' name we ran off tension & stress, anxiety, fear, rejection and fear of it, self-rejection, anger, resentment, rage, discouragement, low body self image, attention deficit disorder, confusion and five imbalance spirits; chemical, biochemical, thyroid, metabolic and hormonal. Trauma and loneliness were also driven off. Finally, we spoke again to HIV and AIDS spirits and again the tingling came on his body. Deliverance and release occurred that he could feel. And, there was a new hope of healing!

One of our favorite radio hosts lost a daughter in her thirties from AIDS. She was infected through blood transference not through her lifestyle. What can you say? Happily, she was a Christian.

In our first book, "God Heals Today", we chronicle a heavily-documented case of the healing of AIDS. It will provide encouragement for anyone suffering with the disease or aware of a suffering friend.

Chiropracty

Marta and her husband were driving east on a vacation. Then it happened. Marta's coffee cup tipped over and very hot coffee poured on to her legs.

The result was extreme pain and second-degree burns. Over a month later, Marta was rubbing on ointment several times a day.

She also had existing liver and kidney problems, plus a neck that bothered her from time to time. How would God heal His daughter? Through Heavenly chiropracty.

Relatives had Marta stand. Her feet were apart. Any spirit of infirmity was cast off the pelvis and the pelvis (hip) was commanded to relax and rotate into the proper alignment. Hands were laid lightly on the area - all in the name of Jesus Christ.

For about an hour, the Spirit moved Marta. Side to side, then front to back. Later, more movements came, including upper-body wiggling , shaking of hands, arms and forearms. More noticeable swaying was part of the divine therapy.

Marta felt better and better. Lighter and lighter. The next afternoon, she felt "good". Pain in the head/neck was non-existent. Her legs were better. Liver and kidneys were improved. God had performed chiropracty as no man could do.

About a week later, Marta wrote to us. The burns on her legs were so healed that she no longer had to apply ointment and bandages several times a day.

Flu comes in a variety of styles, viral and unpleasant any way you look at it. This winter it broke out in the Chicago area and I was caught. Unfortunately, I didn't start rebuking soon enough, so I had some fever for about three days. Happy to say, I did get on the ball and the name of Jesus and things got better. Shows we all miss it sometimes and it's never too late to start and keep on swinging.

Sally missed a lot in life. In her late thirties, she had been in several accidents, automobile and work-place-related. She could use one more back surgery, but there was a 90% chance of losing her life under the knife. Not a very sanguine outlook. In pain from time to time, no feeling in part of her legs, Sally was missing much of life's pleasure.

Additionally, at the time of her deliverance and healing, she had for about four days been seeing double in one eye. On top of that, one of her parents had died just weeks earlier. And - Sally had emotional problems for which she had been medicated. Although she was both bright and articulate, working regularly could pose problems and had limitations.

Over a period of less than three hours, Jesus Christ freed Sally of almost everything that had bound her. And, she felt like a new person. Here's what happened.

As often, the first enemy to be driven out was fear.Then came pre-natal rejection (with a strong release). Following came inherited, residual and childhood spirits of rejection (each manifested separately). Then followed spirits of fear of rejection and self-rejection (both areas included pre-natal, childhood, residual and inherited spirits).

Sally's mother had divorced her father very early on. As a result , she had to and did lose spirits of abandonment and fear of it. The abandonment spirits revealed (for the first time in our experience) a spirit of babyhood abandonment. This was revealed to Sally by the Holy Spirit so it could be driven out.

Terror, dread, panic and trauma left. Many pre-natal, childhood, inherited and residual spirits bit the dust in the areas of hopelessness and frustration.Spirits of suicide, bitterness, resentment and others left. Self-mutilation, inadequacy and fear of it departed.

A background of parental control evidenced when an inherited spirit of control was driven out. Anxiety, stress and tension left. Several times during deliverance, a spirit of deafness came on Sally, to keep her from hearing Faye and I. This had to be dealt with and was.

At the age of thirteen, she had gone to a concert with a warlock and spent the evening (without any relations) with him. The Holy Spirit brought this to mind so we would cast out spirits of spell, witchcraft and spell and warlock trauma. Although Sally is attractive, she gave up a spirit of low body self image.

Among other spirits, Sally was delivered from pre-natal fear of dying, attention deficit disorder and homophobia. Plus a variety of imbalance spirits.

Years of deep resentment toward her natural father left when Sally forgave him and asked God to forgive her.

Faye checked and we determined one leg was shorter than the other. This grew out and part of Sally's back pain left. When hands were laid on her pelvis in the name of Jesus, she felt a tingling. The Lord moved her body around and the Spirit of God moved up from her toes to the upper part of her body.

As a result, not only did pain leave, but areas of her legs which had lost feeling long ago came to life. Now, she could walk freely and pain-free. Years of the canker worm had come to an end.

And - with the heavy anointing present, spirits of manic depression and schizophrenia also manifestly departed. It was awesome.

For the frosting on her cake, after Sally was anointed

with oil, the double vision disappeared.

Then for the cherry on the whipped cream, she received the Baptism in the Holy Spirit with the evidence of speaking in tongues. (Mark 16:17)

At the end of just a part of one Sunday afternoon, Sally was set free and felt like it. Long and traumatic and frustrating years had come to an end. Old things had indeed passed away! (2 Cor.5:17). In fact, just a few weeks later, Sally told us she was able to go back to work. Her life was on the move!

TTP

Chances are you've never heard of Carol Spolnik. But the medical profession has. She suffered from one of the world's very rare diseases - and was blessed by a very rare healing from that disease. Here's the story.

The disease is Thrombotic Thrombocytopenic Purpura. A mouthful of a name - and a dreaded disease. It's a condition characterized by a lower than normal number of blood platelets that results in bleeding and easy bruising. Causes can include drug reaction and diseases of the blood-forming tissues. Chances of recovery are at least as rare as the disease. There is a 75% probability of death and of all of those cases, just one percent don't relapse and die within three years. In 1991, only 111 people in the United States had TTP.

It was in 1991 that Carol went into the hospital. She felt miserable, was bleeding internally. When the disease was diagnosed, her doctors planned to replace all of her blood. This surprising disease was of course a tremendous shock to to the 32-year-old young lady and her family.

However, God was preparing to move in. Karen Andreasen, a close and longtime friend of Carol's, visited her and prayed for her. Then a strange thing happened. Karen, planning to drive from the hospital to a specific location, without meaning to, drove home. When she got out of the car, my wife, Faye, was working in our front yard across the street, which was uncommon for her.

Karen asked for prayer for Carol.And later that day, Faye

and I prayed, taking authority over satanic spirits in the name of Jesus Christ.

On that day, or the next one, the disease was found to be arrested. Carol's blood cells stopped dying. Her red blood count moved up until it finally was even higher than the norm.

One month after the prayer, Carol was released from the hospital. She was miraculously healed. Today, she's healthy, works, sings in her church choir and leads a normal active life. She and her husband have just celebrated the fifth anniversary of her divine healing.

After that, what do you say, except that the Lord is good, and, as Psalm 118 tells us, His mercy does endure forever. And - even the rarest terminal diseases must leave in the mighty name of Jesus Christ!

Karl wrote many reports at work. His hand and wrist were hurting. That's no fun five days a week. But relief was at hand. At a bible study, we commanded that spirit of carpal tunnel syndrome to leave. It was major in the healing. Karl did walk out that night with virtually all pain gone. (He had practiced his hand writing position after the deliverance.)

When, some weeks later, he reported much of that pain had returned, one of us again rebuked the problem and it again departed. We reminded Karl what to do if the devil tried to return to his wrist and hand. Take authority over the situation in the name of Jesus!

Are single men living alone often poor housekeepers? We haven't seen any survey results, but we could make an educated guess.

Harvey fitted into that category, and he didn't deny it. But he was ready for help. And he got it. A spirit of poor housekeeping and then one of procrastination were cast out. Harvey noticed a difference. Hopefully, his apartment became equally shaped up.

Sue Moellering made a costly misstep. She missed a stair and broke two bones in her lower left leg. Also, a chip-

came off of a lower bone. In addition, here was a line fracture under one knee. Not only was Sue hurting, but she heard the doctor state he would probably have to put in a pin in that leg, to remain after the cast was removed.

One evening, Sue's son prayed for her and much of the pain left. Then, a fellow Christian prayed on the phone and the Lord continued the good work He had begun. Spirits of fracture, inflammation, arthritis and pain were commanded out of her. Muscles, ligaments, nerves and tendons were told- to relax and align properly.

Sue something move in the inside of her calf. Almost all of the pain left her - and she felt the power of God, first on her face, then down the front of her body. Can God operate under a cast? You bet.

At a later date, her doctor changed his mind. Sue wouldn't need that pin in her leg after all.

Victory in Jesus. It's occurring minute after minute - most likely right in your city or town. Why not join the rising tide?

Specifics for success

"whatever you shall bind on earth
shall be bound in heaven"
(Matt.16:19 & 18:18)

Why do so many get healed and don't stay healed? Why do so many get delivered and lose all or part of their Jesus-given freedom?

Tanya called with a multitude of problems. People seemed to take advantage of her, lie to her, reject and minimize her, walk all over her. She had been delivered from quite a few spirits, had received help from capable ministries. But, based on the deliverance she received from us, she had lost most of what had been gained in earlier sessions. Why?

She didn't know how to stand or she wasn't using the knowledge she had - at least not often enough. Her downward trend as a loser had continued. Many old enemies had reentered and were negatively affecting her life.

In most cases, we believe, the same devilish group of spirits that lay sickness and/or emotional disease on someone will try to return and do it again.,

Pastor John McCall worked with a well-known healing evangelist in the 1970s. Much too often, when he'd call someone after the healing meetings to get testimonies, the healees were sick or infirm once more. They'd been healed under a powerful anointing, but in their livingrooms and bedrooms, they needed their own faith and the knowledge of how to fight off enemy counterattacks. Without it, not only were healings lost but ammunition was provided for scoffers who claimed these people weren't healed in the first place. It was a sham or mass auto-suggestion of some sort, they proclaimed.

When we talked to Pastor McCall recently, he told us he

teaches weekly on how to keep your healing. This made three facts clear to us. First, many people must be getting healed in his church, or he wouldn't have to teach the subject as often. Second, a bunch of these people was probably getting reafflicted. And third, he realizes how vital it is for his sheep to know how to raise their hackles of authority and not get shorn again.

Jesus warns us in Luke 11:26 that the evil spirits will try to return to the house from which they were ejected. We have to be ready, not paranoid or fearful, but as the apostle Peter advises in 1 Peter 5:8 about our prowling adversary, "resist him, firm in the faith". Notice the two parts to that statement: (1) resist and (2) be firm, not wishy-washy in our faith.

Anxiety, tension, stress and a driving spirit are constantly attacking me or getting on me. I find I have to be constantly vigilant, rebuking them in the name of Jesus. And when I do get into action, I can feel the difference.

There was a lady in a nursing home from whom we cast out a spirit of arthritis on at least six occasions. It would leave, and then when the lady was without help, it would return.

But one Saturday afternoon, this elderly resident informed us she didn't need prayer against arthritis, she was handling the problem herself. And she was, all you had to do was look at her and listen to her. She had learned how to maintain her victory - and it showed!

Nada didn't like the bickering, swearing and fighting that went on among members of her family. After work, she'd usually arrive in the house after the others. Tired, she didn't appreciate the contention and short fuses. Bible-wise, Nada had an answer. Bind in the name of Jesus. So, as she was driving home, she'd take authority over key spirits. She bound spirits of murder, anger, contention, strife. She would also bind negative words and thoughts. Then, she loosed good words and thoughts.

Good report. The atmosphere was more calm, less explosive, more pleasant. Work day after work day, Nada kept the victory the Lord had given her . In Him, there is no darkness at all! (1 John 1:5)

Now, a little advice from someone who's been there - and back.

Shortly after I went through a deliverance session many years ago, I heard of two vital considerations for staying free. The first is -

Be Positive!

Knowing who we are in Christ and what He's done for us by laying down His life and suffering even in hell because He and the Father love us so much - this should help keep us from putting ourselves down and letting the devil walk all over us.

Rejection, inadequacy, unworthiness, depression, discouragement, self-pity and inability are not included in God's picture of us. He says we can do all things through Christ (Phil. 4:19), prospering in whatever we do (Psalm 1:4), more than conquerors (Rom. 8:37), with the joy of the Lord as our strength (Neh. 8:10). Negativism and defeatism aren't joyful and they make us weak - little engines who couldn't instead of could.

So - let's be positive, see ourselves as God's word does, and refuse anything to the contrary. It's true we aren't to think of ourselves more highly than we should. (Rom. 12:3). But that doesn't say we shouldn't esteem ourselves highly. God does. So, we should be "bringing every thought into captivity to the obedience of Christ" (2 Cor. 10:5 KJV). We should focus on the good things (Phil. 4:8). After all, as a man thinks in his heart, "so is he". (Prov. 23:7).

Now, a second consideration for staying free after deliverance.

Don't Go Back Into the World

Look at Israel - and don't make the same mistake.

In the desert, the Israelites longed to go back to Egypt and the bad good old days. They didn't trust their miracle-working Deliverer. And they became bigtime losers. They were scared to death of the giants in Canaan and when God said take the land, they shrank back into oh no land.

Consider secular newspapers, magazines, TV, radio an- movies - and now the internet. Pretty much "having no hope and without God in the world". (Eph. 2:12) Filled with swearing, suggestive sex, violence - often putting down families, especially fathers - with virtually no mention of Jesus Christ. No wonder you so seldom get good news and can easily become programmed negatively.

Remember those inane cocktail parties, especially ones where libidos would break loose? The devil's playgrounds.

How about mutual windows at the race the tracks? Look at the compulsive betters pushing their way in to bet. I know, because from time to time I was one of them, fearing the window would close before I could put my money down.

Even more of these dangerous gambling instincts came out in the stock market. Here, I wound up speculating with not-so-large savings account money. I'm not knocking the stock market, but some people should stay out of it. Yes, the devil's tried to lure me back, but with the help of the Holy Spirit I've stayed out for over 18 years.

My wife and I were once theater subscribers. (And I'm not demeaning that, either.) (Our son , the actor, has been on Broadway.) But, look at most of the story lines and many of the songs in musicals. Would you call them edifying, clean and exemplary ?

For many years, I was a baseball fan. A native of Cleveland, I was, of course, an Indian fan. And when the Tribe got hot a few years ago, baseball fever came on me., After all, when has any team won in its division by 29 games?

But, one Wednesday night in 1995, the Indians were either in the playoffs or World Series. We were praying for people after church service and God was performing a mighty miracle over a period of time.It was important that Faye and I stay. Yet, I was antsy, I wanted to move on and see or hear what was left of the game. My heart wasn't where it should have been. Proverbs 4:23 warns "Watch over your heart with all diligence, for from it flow the issues of life".

Is baseball bad? No. A lot of the players have become Christians and say so. But, when you hear a broadcaster comment on a slider who "took out" the second baseman (and could have injured him) to break up a double play, and he mentions that this is the way it goes, something's wrong. And gradually, this kind of worldly thinking can get into us and drive out the word of God.

Michael Jordan is a fantastic basketball player and seems like a good guy. But hey, to some people, even Christians, hasn't he become an idol? Is a Wednesday night Bulls' game featuring Michael and Scotty Pippen more important than a Wednesday night service featuring Jesus Christ?

I know I'm sticking my neck out, but I also know where I've come from - Egypt. Whether it's compulsive gambling, the lure of lurid theater or greed-driven sports, I realize I can't afford to dabble, try to keep one foot in the world and the other in the word of God.

Besides, what can possibly compare with helping Jesus Christ set someone free, or leading someone to Him and making the difference between heaven and hell? Think about it.

Remember, you, Christian, are seated with Jesus Christ in the spirit world, high above your enemies. They are beneath your feet. (Eph. 2:6 & 1:20) Now, keep them there!

The next chapter should be helpful for those who have lost quite a few evil spirits. It provides a modus operandi, with examples, for keeping the enemy at bay rather than on board.

A daily weapon for victory

"To bind their kings with chains and their nobles with fetters of iron" (Psalm 149:8)

When you've been delivered from one, two or three spirits (physical, emotional or both), it's easy to remember what to stand against. It's even easier when you feel that direct, singular attack coming at you. For example, when the devil came back at me with eye floaters, I could see the problem and successfully rebuke in the name of Jesus.

However, after a batch of spirits have departed, you can use extra help against the counterattaack that may even come the day after deliverance or healing. We've noticed that too many times Christians aren't adequately prepared in such cases. Or a couple of weeks later, the enemy has resurfaced and deliverance is again necessary.

What to do?

What Faye and I find helpful is to arm the deliveree with a written list of the spirits that have been expelled. Then, he or she doesn't have to try to remember. List in hand, that persons can bind (or refuse to permit) those spirits daily in the name of Jesus Christ. When used, it's proving an effective method of staying free.

Here's an example of a deliverance that occasioned giving the person a list. Melba was tired and discouraged, depression had crept in. She was occupied in a construction project for her business, and things weren't going well. She wanted prayer.

The following spirits were ejected in the following order. She felt a release with each of them.

tension & stress	self-rejection
anxiety	inadequacy
fear	fear of inadequacy

depression
discouragement
rejection
fear of rejection
low body self image
anger
resentment

After the deliverance, which didn't take long, Melba felt considerably better. To help her maintain that, we suggested she get a pen or pencil and dictated the list over the phone. We also recommended she bind or rebuke those spirits daily.

In the case of an in-person deliverance, Faye usually notes the spirits that manifestly left during the process and gives a readable copy to the person involved. The list is in order of expulsion. This can be important, if certain spirits were blocking the casting out of other spirits.

Twila still had an upper respiratory infection after two weeks. Her voice sounded heavy, coldish. She also worked in media, with accompanying stresses.

Jesus delivered her from more than the upper respiratory infection that night. Here, in order, is the list.

stress & tension
(more relaxed)
anxiety
inherited worry (parental)
inherited rejection (mom
put down by alcoholic dad)
inherited fear of rejection
inherited & residual self-rejection
inherited inadequacy & fear of it
depression (definitely lighter)
discouragement
jealousy
inherited anger
inherited & residual chemical
imbalance
inherited & residual
imbalance
metabolism imbalance, inherited
ADD (Difficulty
concentrating)
narcolepsy (sleepy
at wrong times)
insomnia
driving spirit
inherited dr. spirit
residual driving
spirit
residual restlessness
(after she rebuked it)
doubt (strong)
fear of mother dying
inherited rebellion
inherited perverse
(headache now gone)
inherited self-pity
residual self-pity

residual & otherwise
hormonal imbalance
low body self image
self-pity
scoliosis (back pain left)

AND THESE PHYSICAL TORMENTORS:

strep throat
inherited strep throat
residual strep throat
chronic fatigue syndrome
strong release with chills
grew out left leg

At end of session:
voice normal
she felt better

Faye dictated the above list to Twila and suggested she bind those spirits daily. Twila has followed up and kept free of many of her enemies.

Sylvia was unhappy. Understandably. She had been rejected in a part of her community. Although physical problems were not her reasons for accepting help, she did have them: chest pain, arthritis, constantly drippy nose. Her case shows how important the order of deliverance can be. It also reveals how a sizeable clan of spirits can weave a web and hold a victim captive.

To better understand what follows, you should know that Sylvia suffered abuse and rejection from childhood and she had been raped. Improper overtures were also made to her when she was a child.

Now, the deliverance.

As we often do, we began with tension & stress, then anxiety, fear, and rejection. This time, there was no response. Now we suspected blocking spirits.And that proved to be the case.When we commanded rape/trauma to leave in Jesus' name, it did. The same happened with residual rape/trauma fear. We had no further success until a spirit of suicide was cast out - and Sylvia cried. Then came:

grief
sadness
low body self image
childhood rejection
childhood inadequacy
inherited chemical imbalance
" thyroid imbalance
" metabolic imbalance
" hormonal imbalance
CHEST PAIN GONE

childhood fear of men	inherited rheumatoid arthritis
childhood abandonment	sinusitis, allergic rhinitis &
fear of abandonment	catarrh
childhood anxiety	bronchitis
residual anxiety	childhood lust
stress & tension	anger
shame	bitterness
childhood shame	confusion
childhood depression	FELT MUCH BETTER
residual depression	

At this point, we prayed for PEACE and God sent it strongly.

Time for deliverance - roughly 50 minutes

Could Sylvia remember all the spirits she had been delivered from? Of course not. So, when the session was completed, we dictated the list of spirits to her. And we advised she refuse them daily and when needed, in the name of Jesus. In spiritual warfare, prevention should always follows cure.

A variety of demonic attacks bombarded Mina in the course of a week. Death in the family. Emotional disquiet. Falling several times at work, for no apparent reason. She called for the Lord's assistance just prior to the funeral. Here's the order of deliverance:

root of bitterness	discouragement
fear	inherited ADD
fear of the future	confusion
anxiety	hormonal imbalance
stress & tension	dizziness
anger	myasthenia gravis
rage	(above two often together)
hostility	heart infirmity
depression	palpitations

By the time ADD (attention deficit disorder) had left, Mina felt peace. After myasthenia gravis departed, there was more peace. When the final spirit had gone, she reported being "even more relaxed".

Mina had been rebuking some of the spirits she was aware of, but this had been a demonic group, project - and on-going success comes from rebuking all of the spirits on a regular basis. We listed the spirits for her and suggested she take authority over them daily or even more often. Mina is a fighter and she'll do battle in the name of Jesus!

The following healing could also go (along with others) in the Emotional Blockers chapter. Missy was healed physical after emotional spirits left.

Her ankle and foot hurt, especially when she walked. Soreness was addressed and there was a little relief. Pain was cast out many times, indicating many such spirits were resident. And there was improvement. More reaction came when osteoarthritis (which had apparently sneaked in, as it will often do) left. Bursitis and another spirit of pain departed. Then, muscular tension.

Next came the ejection of emotional spirits - in the following order (some physical spirits were interspersed):

anxiety	fear of future
fretting	pain (once more)
frustration	inherited circulation
depression	sympathy
doubt	frustration
despondency	sympathetic pain
despair	

Sympathetic pain was s major blocker. Missy had a close relative who had a somewhat similar physical problem. The sympathetic had most likely entered when Missy was overly concerned. So, she could be attacked successfully. When this last spirit left, the remainder of the pain left her. She could walk briskly around the room - with no pain!

Yes, she has the list of enemies to bind (refuse) daily or as often as needed. She can avoid a recurrence in the name of Jesus.

How long is it necessary to run the list? Just once daily, or more often each day? That would depend on the individual, we believe. Some find that the list can be shortened considerably as time goes on. In time, it may not be necessary as one builds up on the word of God and tries to avoid problem areas or change attitudes.

How to Win

"The Lord is with you, O valiant warrior. Go in this your strength and deliver" (Judges 6:12 & 14)

If you're a born-again Christian, here's what you do.

Prevention

At the first sign of a mental or physical incursion, or a counterattack after deliverance, pull out the key of binding (or refusing to permit). (Matt. 16:19) Remember, Prov.18:10 promises, "The name of the Lord is a strong tower; the righteous runs into it and is safe." Also, recall that in John 17:11 (NIV) Jesus prayed we would be kept safe by the power of His name. He has given us His name to use!

Specifically, let's say you're starting to feel anxious. Simply speak to that mountain as follows: "Spirit of anxiety, I refuse you in the name of Jesus." If you like, you can add an appropriate scripture such as Jesus' injunction not to be anxious. (Luke 12:22)

Perhaps fear is attacking, you say, "Spirit of fear, I refuse you in the name of Jesus. " Again, you can add scripture such as Psalm 118:6, " The Lord is son my side; I will not fear" (KJV). Including scripture is helpful, but not necessary.

On the physical side, if you're starting to get a headache, here's the remedy. Say to it, "Spirit of headache, I refuse you in the name of Jesus". For a head cold, "Spirit of head cold, I refuse you, in the name of Jesus". Etc., just change the name of the spirit to fit the attacker.

Whatever the symptoms are, keep refusing them in the

name of Jesus until they leave or you get a release in your spirit.

Cure

If a particular problem, or set of problems, has been around a while and has a hold on you (or someone else), you must loose it. Don't loose (or cast out) from a non-Christian. That person can't use the authority of Jesus to prevent the spirit from returning and bringing others with it. (Matt. 12:43-45)

To loose, as with binding (refusing), speak to the specific mountain, (flu, anxiety or whatever). The problem exists, but but the causing spirit must leave when you command it to.

In every case, binding or loosing, speak as if you mean it. Jesus spoke with authority and demons didn't hang around. You should do the same!

Binding and loosing are not exact sciences. I can't tell you how many times you'll have to speak to those mountains. Your faith and the strength of the spirit can be involved. Also, there could be blocking spirits, (see Chapter 7) that must be handled first. If you're not sure what's blocking, ask the Lord. He doesn't want you to be ignorant or go on suffering.

Often, physical or emotional spirits may be inherited, be pre-natal, come from childhood or be long-residing. If that seems to be the case, try speaking to those spirits specifically. (An inherited or generational spirit can go back at least four generations. Ex. 20:5)

Another possible blocker is unforgiveness. If you're holding anything against anyone, even if it's their fault, God says you must forgive (Mark 11:25 & 26) and ask God to forgive you for not forgiving. Also, if you have any other unconfessed sin, confess it to God and get on with the deliverance. If you're delivering someone else, the same procedure can apply.

Sometimes, you may be where you can't speak aloud. Don't worry about it. Speak in your mind. It will work. God is a deliverer not a legalist.

Finally, be aware of I Peter 5:8, "Your adversary, the devil prowls around like a roaring lion, seeking someone to devour, but resist him, firm in your faith".

Victory over every sin, sickness and pain is constantly in your grasp. God has provided a way out. Go for it - in the name of the Lord! These are the last of the last days and Jesus is shaping up His people for victory after victory, soul after soul.

Be the winner God made you to be!

Healthy bodies are healthy choices

"Or do you not know your body is a temple of the Holy Spirit" (I Corinthians 6:19)

Christian, God lives inside of you. And he expects you and I to keep His houses clean and up to snuff. He's the owner and we're the lessees. So the condition of our frames and furnishings is important to the Lord.

Let's face it, we live in a sugar-and-spice, not beanss-and-rice age. Fatty foods fill supermarket shelves, but they don't have to fill us. We can control our cholesterol, etc, by looking at labels and watching what we eat. I'm far from being a diet specialist. My wife, though, is home economist and knows whereof she buys, prepares and cooks our cuisine.

Most experts, including the U.S. government, like that word "balanced". Too much of anything can glut us, and if it includes enough of the wrong stuff, it can glut our arteries as well.Today, fruits and vegetables and whole grains are making a comeback. Many of us are eating lighter and feeling and looking the same way.

Unqualified as I am in this area, I'm addressing it, in part, because on radio interviews, I'm often asked about it. One Christian hostess now has two shows - one on the supernatural power of God, and the other on making wise natural choices.

I do know that almost as soon as I became a Christian, the Lord led me to abandon sugars and red meats. Since those days, nearly 19 years ago, my energy level has been higher and maintained longer and the prostate problem He healed has not returned. I'm in better shape to serve him to a greater extent.

Speaking of red meats, tasty though they may be, I did learn something from my then-in-high-school son. John took a health or cooking class in which he found out that red meats were considered a possible cause of prostate cancer. And when I'm somewhere that has steak, hamburger, veal or ham on the menu, it's healthy for me to remember that information - even chew on it. Especially when my dad, who ate red meats just about always except on fridays, died from cancer that began in the prostate.

After my salvation, the Lord did a remarkable sovereign work. Not only was I content without red meat, but he took away from this once sugarholic any desire for sweets. I could gaze at a luscious-looking cake without batting a taste bud. Of course, as time went on, the protective blanket came off and, I've had to stand on my own appetite. And I do admit I've sometimes fallen. But I've pretty much stayed on track - and so has my weight and energy.

Alcohol? It is, or should be, common knowledge that a major percentage of traffic deaths are alcohol-related. I worked as an election judge in the November, 1996 general election. At the polling place, a middle-aged voter told us her husband had been killed by a drunk driver - and she was hospitalized from that accident for six months.The lady was very bitter thaat the drunk driver was still out there. Multiply that kind of tragedy to the nth degree and you're looking at heartache unfathomable.

Years ago, I would sometimes have a bottle or two of beer after bowling or at a party with my wife. Driving home one night, I realized the car I was piloting was weaving down the road. We, and/or others could have been killed. After that, my occasional light drinking came to a halt. Who needs it?

Consider families and marriages ripped apart by alcoholic spirits. Imagine the lives affected through generations - in addition ato the drinking that brings abuse and provides a cowardly hiding place from responsibility. Not to mention the shame, guilt and shattered self-esteem of the drinker.

We sometimes pray for people caught in that demonic web. It seems to be as prevalent and it is destructive. Elsewhere in this book, we cite a case of an adult who picked up a childhood spirit of alcohol from drinking with his dad at age 14. Bon vivant and good cheer? Pain, depression, destruction and death!

Born again - the Why and How

"Truly, truly, I say to you, unless one is born again, he cannot see the kingdom of God.." (John 3:3)

Jesus makes it clear. He says in Verse 5, "Unless one is born of water (physical birth) and of the Spirit (spiritual birth), he cannot enter the kingdom of God".

There are only two spiritual kingdoms in the world - the kingdom of Satan ("the god of this world", II Cor. 4:4 KJV) and the kingdom of God, which is in this world, but not of it. (John 18:36) When we are born again, or born from above, this spiritual birth delivers us out of "the domain of darkness" and transferred "to the kingdom of His beloved Son". When you ask Jesus Christ to come into your heart to be your Lord (not just "the" Lord), believing God raised Him from the dead, He enters in and you immediately enter into the kingdom of God!

That's becoming "born again".

And as soon as you enter His kingdom, all of God's promises in the Bible are for you. (II Cor. 1:19)

Not only do these promises include eternal life with God and Jesus, but also everything necessary for a more abundant life. (John 10:10) And that includes delegated authority from Jesus Christ to refuse to permit or to cast out the evil spirits that cause every sickness and pain, physical and emotional.

Getting into this wonderful kingdom of God is surprisingly easy. According to the Book of Romans, Chapter 10, Verse 9, "if you confess (say) with your mouth Jesus as Lord, and in believe in your heart God raised Him from the dead, you shall be saved".

So, if you don't already know Jesus Christ as your Lord and Savior (I went to church for years and didn't know Him), here's a simple way to do it. Just say aloud the following prayer -

"Lord Jesus, I believe in my heart that God raised you from the dead. I ask you now to come into my heart and be my Lord and Savior. And I say with my mouth. "Jesus Christ is my Lord."

If you prayed that prayer, welcome to the family of God! You've become one of His beloved children - and He'll never leave you or forsake you.

And He's also waiting to help you achieve victory over sickness and pain!

More help for winning

"Every fact is to be confirmed by the testimony of two or three witnesses." (2 Cor. 13:1)

More and more fine books are coming out on deliverance and healing. In just the past three years, many of those in the list below have been published. There's much to be gleaned and discovered from these books. Certainly, in these last of the last days, we can use all the ammunition we can find. The latter rain seems to be falling and it can increase as more of God's vessels are prepared to move in the knowledge and authority Jesus Christ has given us.

Authority in Three Worlds	Charles Capps
The Believer's Authority	Kenneth Hagin
The Bondage Breaker	Neil Anderson
Christian, Set Yourself Free	G. & S. Powell
Defeating Dark Angels	Charles H. Kraft
Deliverance From Evil Spirits	Francis MacNutt
Deliver Us From Evil	Don Basham
Demons and Deliverance	Frank Hammond
Demons The Answer Book	Lester Sumrall
God Heals Today	Chuck Schiappacasse
God's Health Care Plan	Chuck Schiappacasse
Healing Handbook	C. & F. Hunter
Healing Promises	K. & G. Copeland
Healing Through Deliverance #2	Peter Horrobin
Healing Through Spiritual War...	Peggy Scarborough
Jesus Taught Me To Cast Out	Norvel Hayes
Medicine For the Mind	Steve Sampson
The Name of Jesus	Kenneth Hagin
Pigs In the Parlor	F. & I. Hammond
Released to Reign	Charles Trombley
Spiritual Warfare	Michael Harper
Spiritual Warfare	Richard Ing
Strategic Spiritual Warfare	Beeson & Hussey

25. Victorious Reading

Victory In Spiritual Warfare......... Gary Whetstone
You Can Hear the Voice of God.... Steve Sampson

Teachers are placed in the body of Christ for the equipping of the saints for the work of service. (Eph. 4:12) There is no doubt that all of us who are Christians (and therefore saints) can use the equipment the Lord is providing us.

The latter rain is to bring in the harvest of souls. As God pours it out among and through us, we will be better able to not only free ourselves and our brothers - but we'll have more of what it takes to move out in the power evangelism that, as in the early rain over 1900 years ago, can again turn our world upside down for Jesus Christ!

AFTERWORD

In the great majority of incidents related in this book, we've used pseudonyms. However, we can definitely assure you the healings/deliverances did occur. When first and last names are used, these are the real names of the persons involved.

Can we guarantee you health and healing if you follow the precepts, scriptures and suggestions in the book? Of course not. But we have related what we've experienced and received from reliable sources - and you will find the contents very biblically-based.

The opportunity of working with the Head of the church (Mark 16:20) to get free, set free and stay free is available to every born-again Christian. You don't have to have a special ministry or ministry gift.. When you have Jesus Christ in your heart and you command evil spirits to go in His name, they must comply. Remember, Psalm 149:9 (KJV) assures you "this honour have all His saints".

Now - start setting the captives free!

If you have experienced physical or emotional healing through the use of the authority of believers - or if you know of someone who has - please write to us at *God Heals Today, P.O. Box 214, Glenview , IL.* Or call 1-800-760-BOOK.

INDEX

<u>at the name of Jesus, EVERY KNEE SHOULD BOW</u>

(Phil. 2:10)

Chapter 21 includes listing of some spirits not indicated above.